STRATEGIC SKILLS FOR PUBLIC HEALTH PRACTICE SERIES

Data-Informed Decision Making

USING DATA TO BUILD CONSENSUS AND ALIGN PRIORITIES

For access to digital chapters,
visit the APHA Press bookstore (www.apha.org).

Strategic Skills for Public Health Practice Series
Series Editors: Michael Fraser, PhD, MS, and Brian C. Castrucci, DrPH

1. *Systems and Strategic Thinking*
2. *Policy Engagement*
3. *Resource Management and Finance*
4. *Community Engagement*
5. *Advancing Equity and Justice*
6. *Effective Communication*
7. *Change Management*
8. *Data-Informed Decision Making*
9. *Cross-Sectoral Partnerships*

STRATEGIC SKILLS FOR PUBLIC HEALTH PRACTICE

SERIES

Data-Informed Decision Making

USING DATA TO BUILD CONSENSUS AND ALIGN PRIORITIES

Chad Abresch, PhD

Carol Gilbert, PhD, MS

Regina Idoate, PhD

Ellen Kerns, PhD, MPH

Aislinn Rookwood, PhD

APHA PRESS

AN IMPRINT OF AMERICAN PUBLIC HEALTH ASSOCIATION

American Public Health Association
800 I Street, NW
Washington, DC 20001-3710
www.apha.org

Georges C. Benjamin, MD, MACP, Executive Director

Printed and bound in the United States of America
Book Production Editor: Keira McCarthy
Typesetting: The Charlesworth Group
Cover Design: Alan Giarcanella
Printing and Binding: Sheridan Books

Library of Congress Cataloging-in-Publication Data

Names: Abresch, Chad, author. | Gilbert, Carol (Writer on public health), author. | Idoate, Regina, author. | Kerns, Ellen, author. | Rookwood, Aislinn, author.
Title: Data-informed decision-making : using data to build consensus and align priorities / authors Chad Abresch, PhD, Carol Gilbert, PhD, MS, Regina Idoate, PhD, Ellen Kerns, PhD, MPH, Aislinn Rookwood, MPH.
Description: Washington, DC : American Public Health Association, [2024] | Includes bibliographical references and index. | Summary: "This book arms public health professionals with the skills needed to find and extract as much information as possible from existing data sources, evaluate the limits of our factual knowledge, and improve analyses by including communities in both analysis and programmatic decision making"-- Provided by publisher.
Identifiers: LCCN 2024028384 (print) | LCCN 2024028385 (ebook) | ISBN 9780875533568 (paperback) | ISBN 9780875533575 (adobe pdf)
Subjects: LCSH: Public health--Decision making--Data processing. | Public health--Decision making.
Classification: LCC RA427 .A27 2024 (print) | LCC RA427 (ebook) | DDC 362.10285--dc23/eng/20241112
LC record available at https://lccn.loc.gov/2024028384
LC ebook record available at https://lccn.loc.gov/2024028385

To all who work tirelessly to improve community health—public health professionals, community leaders, and engaged citizens. Meaningful and lasting solutions emerge when we unite scientific rigor with community wisdom and action. Together, we transform data into understanding and understanding into decisions that drive innovation to improve health and well-being.

Contents

Strategic Skills for Public Health Practice Series Introduction

Over the last 15 years, governmental public health professionals and partners nationwide have worked to define core competencies, essential services, and foundational capabilities of the public health.[1,2,3] Central to all these efforts is the public health workforce—the practitioners who work in local, state, territorial, tribal, and federal public health agencies to prevent disease and protect and promote the health of the public.

The governmental public health workforce is diverse and comprised of many technical specialties and professions. These professional identities have shaped public health practice and formed categories of work that comprise the organizational chart most governmental public health agencies utilize, such as maternal and child health, environmental health, epidemiology and surveillance, communicable disease control, administration and finance, school health, and several others.

These categories have served public health well by helping organize work and allowing for professionalization and leadership development within specific areas. Over 21 national professional associations represent categorical or function areas within state and territorial health departments alone, not to mention peer groups and affinity groups that are part of the Association of State and Territorial Health Officials and other allied organizations such as the National Association of County and City Health Officials, the Big Cities Health Coalition, CityMatCH (urban maternal and child health programs), the National Environmental Health Association, and others.

These specialty designations have also led to fragmentation within agencies at a time when government is attempting to align more nimbly to meet the needs of the jurisdictions they serve. Few public health professionals have formal training in the skills needed to successfully adapt their work to navigate these changes, especially the strategic skills needed to position their work to meet contemporary public health challenges that require inter- and intra-agency collaboration for success. For example, the pressures and challenges imposed on the public health ecosystem and its workers by the COVID-19 pandemic illustrate the urgency of preparing the public health workforce not just for technical challenges but also for strategic and adaptive challenges posed by novel health threats that require an "all of government" approach to resolve.

Several external forces in recent years, including the movement from Public Health 2.0 to Public Health 3.0 and the six-year-long, three-phased Public Health Workforce Interests and Needs Survey, have either advocated for or implied the need for complementing the workforce's existing discipline-specific expertise with developing a set of strategic skills.

In 2017, the de Beaumont Foundation spearheaded the development of the National Consortium for Public Health Workforce Development comprised of public health leaders from 34 national partner organizations representing a variety of disciplines and settings nationwide. The Consortium was established "to communicate the needs of the front-line public health worker to national partners and funders."[4]

By consensus, the Consortium identified the following nine "indispensable, high-performance skills applicable to the entire public health workforce regardless of specialty or discipline."[5]

- Systems and strategic thinking
- Change management
- Effective communication
- Data-informed decision making
- Community engagement
- Justice, equity, diversity, and inclusion
- Resource management and finance
- Policy engagement
- Cross-sectoral partnerships

These strategic skills are needed by specialty-specific, technical experts in order to realize the multisector, cross-cutting visionary leadership needed today. The Consortium's "call to action" paper asserted this challenge to public health educators: "While maintaining excellence in core scientific disciplines continues to be a priority, developers and deliverers of public health education and training need to act in new and different ways if the governmental public health workforce is to gain competency in the strategic skills needed throughout the entire public health workforce."[5]

Creating these "new and different ways" of building public health workforce competencies in the strategic skills should be a priority for academic programs, professional associations, and public health partners nationwide. This Strategic Skills Series presents a new way to expand the education and training of the public health workforce, equipping its members for multisector collaboration to create policies and programs intended to solve real problems.

To develop this series, we have recruited thought leaders and experts to serve as the authors of each volume. The consistent format applied to each book in the series is intended to facilitate the learner's absorption and retention of key concepts and applications. The practice-based objectives of each book in the series are described below:

- **Systems and strategic thinking:** Grasp patterns and relationships to understand systems contributing to public health problems and identify high-impact interventions.
- **Change management:** Scale programs in response to the changing environments and shape core elements that sustain programs in challenge and crisis.
- **Effective communication:** Convey resonant, compelling public health messages to broad audiences—the public, partners, and policymakers.
- **Data-informed decision making:** Leverage, synthesize, and analyze multiple sources of electronic data and use informatics to identify and act on health priorities, population impacts, evidence-based approaches, and health and cost-related outcomes.
- **Community engagement:** Describe the most effective methods of and the beneficial outcomes from engaging communities in promoting health and well-being. Promote the model of equitable distribution of decision-making power.
- **Justice, equity, diversity, and inclusion:** Understand and respond to the changing demographics of the US population and the public health workforce itself. Seek out, listen to, include, and promote underrepresented populations in reaching effective health solutions.
- **Resource management and finance:** Oversee recruitment, acquisition, and retention of the workforce and manage fiscal resources responsibly.
- **Policy engagement:** Address public health concerns and needs and engage effectively with local, state, and federal policymakers and partners.
- **Cross-sectoral partnerships:** Bring together two or more distinct fields (e.g., health care and transportation) for greater impact so that public health professionals can maintain long-term collaborations that combine a unique set of resources, experience, and knowledge to effectively address multifaceted issues (e.g., the social determinants of health).

As we aim to move public health forward to meet the challenges of contemporary practice, we are excited to edit each of these volumes. It is our fervent hope that each of the books in this series represents a significant brick in the foundation of developing your capacity to address today's urgencies as well as tomorrow's opportunities and challenges.

Michael Fraser, PhD, MS
Brian C. Castrucci, DrPH

REFERENCES

1. Public Health Foundation. Core competencies for public health professionals. 2014. Accessed January 22, 2021. http://www.phf.org/programs/corecompetencies/Pages/Core_Competencies_Domains.aspx
2. US Centers for Disease Control and Prevention. 10 essential public health services. 2020. Accessed August 30, 2024. https://www.cdc.gov/public-health-gateway/php/about/index.html

3. Public Health National Center for Innovation. Foundational public health services. 2018. Accessed August 30, 2024. https://phaboard.org/wp-content/uploads/FPHS-Factsheet-2022.pdf
4. de Beaumont Foundation. Building skills for a more strategic public health workforce: a call to action. 2019. Accessed September 26, 2022. https://debeaumont.org/wp-content/uploads/2019/04/Building- Skills-for-a-More-Strategic-Public-Health-Workforce.pdf
5. de Beaumont Foundation. Building skills for a more strategic public health workforce: a call to action. July 18, 2017. Accessed January 22, 2021. https://www.debeaumont.org/news/2017/building-skills-for-a-more-strategic-health-workforce-a-call-to-action

Acknowledgments

We are deeply grateful to the many individuals who helped bring this book to fruition. Special thanks to Dr. Brian C. Castrucci, whose thorough reviews and critical eye challenged us to think more deeply and broadly about the complex interplay between data and community engagement. His insightful feedback markedly strengthened the final manuscript. We are indebted to Maya Ribault for her unwavering support, patience, and consummate professionalism throughout the writing process. Her steady guidance kept us on track while allowing us the space to fully develop our ideas. We thank Dr. Michael Fraser for both the inspiration behind this volume and the invitation to contribute as authors. Most importantly, we are profoundly grateful to the maternal and child health leaders in local health departments across the country who have allowed us to learn alongside them as they work to improve outcomes in their communities. The stories and lessons shared in these pages are drawn from their experiences and dedication to data-informed, community-centered public health practice.

Preface

> **Geri's Story**
>
> As she sipped her coffee, Geri listened to fragments of conversations in small groups around the room. She had just finished presenting a wealth of infant mortality data from her community and, unfortunately, the data did not paint an optimistic picture. When compared nationally, Geri's community ranked toward the bottom in infant mortality. Too many babies were being born prematurely, sleep-related deaths were also too high, and racial inequities in infant survival had not improved significantly in the past decade. Despite the work that needed to be done, Geri felt a sense of relief—the data were finally "out there" and could be used to motivate change.
>
> As a representative of the health department, Geri hoped the data would inform the community members in attendance. She envisioned the group reaching consensus and agreeing to take strategic action. Her presentation seemed to have gone well. The room was attentive, and she noticed various active responses. Eyes lit up as new understandings and implications dawned. Heads nodded, gratified that the data confirmed their thinking. Many were taking notes. These were all good signs. However, she noticed that some people looked skeptical at points.
>
> As conversation began, Geri could hear concerns creeping in. An immigrant rights worker did not trust Geri's numbers on race and ethnicity. A neonatologist felt that Geri's study should have included surrounding counties where many of his preemies and sick babies came from. A young mother doubted that having less than a high school education could cause health problems. There was also anxiety about the changes that might be required. A manager worried about keeping her program funded. An obstetrician knew she couldn't fit another set of screening questions into her office routine. Several more people sat quietly but looked perplexed. Geri began to wonder what she could do to harness the brains in the room and help them reach consensus to move the community forward. How could she provide better data or frame them differently to lead to consensus?

Data can illuminate otherwise murky issues, providing clarity instead of guesswork. Data can be used to evaluate performance, improve efforts, make profits, justify hard decisions, and even settle seemingly impossible disputes. In a diverse group, data can provide a factual foundation on which everyone can agree.

However, data do not always provide clear and definitive answers. For example, think back to an improbable score you witnessed in a sporting event. It may have been amazing, but was it legal? Did it really count? In an earlier era, we had only the opinion of the referee, but as we watch our favorite players and teams today, data pour across the screen constantly, providing evidence we can use to check the accuracy of the referees. We are shown multiple angles in high definition with slow-motion video. However, the analysis often becomes so nuanced that it makes our heads spin and the definitive answer to whether the score was legitimate or not remains elusive. Once again, we find ourselves back in the realm of opinion, forced to accept the interpretation of the referee. Even in this high-tech, well-funded, data-rich situation, "truth" is often not as clear as we wish it to be.

Consider Geri's story. It is a story that the authors have seen play out in communities across the country time and again. In fact, we have frequently helped "Geri" put together her data presentation, assisting her to present the best data possible. If the data aren't explained carefully and thoroughly, her audience may misunderstand and not reach consensus. After all, change can be difficult and in public health, there is always something to dispute.

How can we help Geri and her community do a better job of using data to make decisions? Can Geri be more transparent about the limitations of her data, yet make strong recommendations based only on the available evidence? Can she bring more "truth" to her analysis by involving people with different traditions and perspectives in her selection of data sources, study questions, and analytic methods? Can she more systematically account for biases caused by excluding parts of the population or by missing or messy data elements? Perhaps the most important question is this: What should we do when action needs to be taken, but we don't have all the information, or don't agree on what is true?

Public health decision makers must admit that incontrovertible evidence is seldom available, yet decisions must be made. For too long, we, as public health professionals, have asked too much of data. This book gives public health professionals the necessary skills to find and extract as much information as possible from existing data sources, carefully evaluate the limits of our factual knowledge, and improve our analyses by including communities in both analysis and programmatic decision making. We explore techniques for communicating our data processes and outcomes with the goals of inviting participation, stimulating discussion, questioning assumptions, and reaching a consensus that is informed by what the data do and do not tell us. Each chapter discusses a step in the process and includes considerations for a range of data types. We also discuss opportunities for community input, real-world stories of success and failure, and resources for diving deeper into various topics (see the following figure in the Preface).

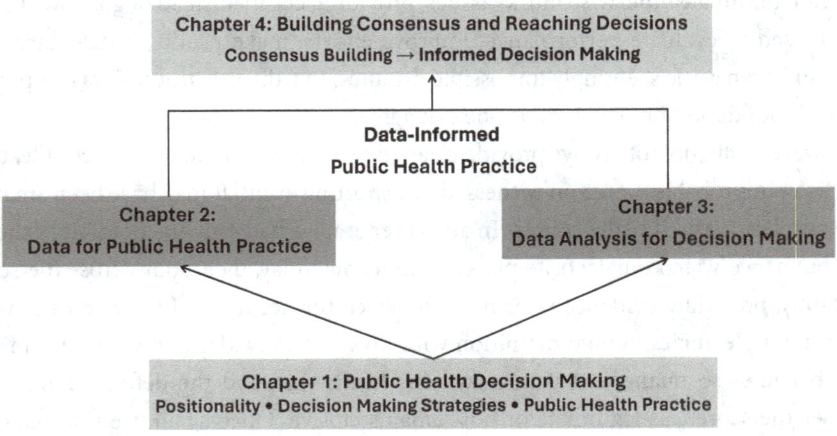

Framework for Data-Informed Decision Making

Chapter 1 addresses the intricacies of public health decision making amid myriad, often competing priorities. How can the public health workforce successfully navigate so many viewpoints? In this context, we introduce the critical concept of positionality, which urges introspection into how our personal backgrounds shape our unique perspectives. Not only do public health professionals need to understand and respect the positionality of community members, but their success depends upon being thoughtful and transparent about their own positionality.

Chapter 2 highlights the importance of using both scientific literature and local data sources for informing public health practice. We discuss various secondary data sources, including population-based surveys, disease surveillance systems, health care data, and place-based data, while acknowledging their advantages, limitations, and potential biases. The chapter also emphasizes the value of collecting primary data through methods like surveys, interviews, focus groups, and observations, as they can provide contextualized information tailored to the community's needs. Additionally, we underscore the significance of addressing potential biases, such as differential response rates, data collection modes, and privacy and data sovereignty concerns, to ensure accurate and representative data for effective public health decision making.

In Chapter 3, we emphasize the importance of a systematic and community-engaged approach to data analysis for effective public health decision making. The chapter outlines five guiding principles: clearly understanding the purpose of the analysis, examining relevant causal relationships, consulting complementary data sources, identifying potential biases, and involving the community. Next, we discuss various considerations for good scientific practice, including understanding the limitations of our data sources, using appropriate denominators, diagramming problems, linking and synthesizing datasets, building new evidence through evaluation, and always partnering with community members. The overarching theme is the need for a rigorous, inclusive, and contextually grounded analytical process that leverages diverse perspectives and data to inform sound public health decisions.

In Chapter 4, we draw on all previous content to address the topic of using data to inform public health decision making. The chapter provides real-world examples of instances where data-informed public health action and the community came into conflict. To address and resolve these frequent conflicts, we propose a set of principles informed by the emotional intelligence literature. Our key point is that effective public health data use is more than just analytic capacity. Instead, it depends on self-awareness and social empathy.

The book finishes with a short conclusion, which stresses that data-informed decision making is crucial for effective public health practice but points out that access to essential data sources remains a significant challenge. In our view, restrictions on data access and use have been rapidly increasing, often hindering health departments from fulfilling their core functions effectively. While data owners have legitimate concerns regarding data security, handling practices, and political sensitivities, excessive restrictions hamper the ability of health departments and their partners to make informed decisions based on the best available evidence. Moving forward, we believe a broader conversation within the public health field is imperative to address data use and access issues, including efficient data use agreement processes that help ensure appropriate data analysis and dissemination and facilitate collaboration with partner organizations to leverage their expertise.

Chad Abresch, PhD
Carol Gilbert, PhD, MS
Regina Idoate, PhD
Ellen Kerns, PhD, MPH
Aislinn Rookwood, PhD

1

Public Health Decision Making

Public health practice is complex and must be responsive to multiple, often divergent, expectations from constituents. Data are powerful and can help public health practitioners respond to constituents in both research and practice. Data should guide the types of questions we ask, the methods we select to answer those questions, and the analytic and dissemination strategies we employ. However, the meaning each of us derives from data differs based on our personal life context—what's known as positionality. As public health professionals, we can improve our effectiveness by becoming clear about our positionality and sharing it with communities as we partner to improve health. This chapter offers a starting point for effective data use by exploring the complexity of public health decision making and presenting an opportunity for readers to understand positionality in their work.

THE COMPLEXITY OF PUBLIC HEALTH PRACTICE

This book is written for the public health workforce, which is defined here as any person whose job involves shaping programs and policies designed to improve the health and well-being of a selected community or population. So, whether you work for a state, local, or tribal public health department, a nonprofit agency, or perhaps as a consultant or a public health ally, this book is for you. We wrote this book because public health decision making is complex, and no easy or singular formula exists for getting it right. The public health workforce is faced with an onslaught of often divergent expectations, including the following:

- Elected officials expect public health activities that are responsive to their administration's agendas and aligned with their political goals and campaign promises.
- Public health project funders establish their own priorities and often require grantees to adhere to published guidelines and specific grant policies.
- Accreditation bodies and federal agencies expect public health activities that are evidence based and that demonstrate careful epidemiological assessments.
- Citizens expect public health activities that reflect their priorities and are planned and delivered using inclusive approaches.

Balancing these often-divergent expectations is a central feature of public health practice. The challenge of "getting it right" is ever present. It does not stop after the needs assessment is complete or a new program is implemented. Making the matter even more complex is the fact that the public health workforce has expectations too. Taking their expectations into account is critical to ensuring that our public health employees feel authentic in the work they do and believe in the possibility of truly making a positive difference. Being able to practice public health in this way helps sustain effort in what is often difficult work and ultimately leads to higher quality and the potential for more positive public health impact.

What about the data? What do the data demand? In a word, nothing. We often speak of data as living, sentient beings. We routinely personify data when we use expressions like, "the data demand action" or "what these data are telling us." These expressions may seem harmless, but they mask an all-too-common public health faux pas—allowing thinly understood data rather than our own sense of purpose and the will of the populations we serve to dictate our actions.

When people say things like "the data demand action," they generally mean they *personally* find the data to be unacceptable and deserving of action. In these instances, the data are serving as their proof—their "Exhibit A"—that something must be done. They may have a strong point. However, it is important to also remember that data (e.g., numbers, facts, stories) are always a limited representation of reality. We do not have data to measure all of what is important, and when we rely on a narrow dataset, it can lead us astray (see Chapter 2). Including diverse types of data like art, contemporary folklore, music, numbers, stories, characters, and caricatures enables us to gain greater clarity into the rich and complex picture of human social existence and how it shapes our patterns of health. One data source should never be the basis for our public health decision making. Similarly, one person's interpretation of the data should not determine our actions. We must listen to community voices from multiple and diverse sectors, blending and balancing their unique input to find an agreeable path toward better health for all.

As wielders of public health data, we must also remember that we hold powerful information capable of eliciting strong emotional responses. The authors of this book have spent their careers sharing data with community groups and have observed the power of data on multiple occasions: "You mean not every community experiences this many infant deaths? What are they doing differently and why didn't we start doing that a long time ago?" As community members grasp specific data points, we have often witnessed tears, outrage, disbelief, and on occasion, enough passion to launch large-scale public health initiatives that endure for a decade or more. Interestingly, there have been many instances when public health workers were caught off guard by the community's response to the data they presented. All this underscores the point: data do not dictate public health action—people do.

We all use data to make meaning, and in turn, we use meaning to shape action. While this may seem simple and self-evident, as public health professionals, it is an important truth to keep front and center because it reminds us that each person will see the data through their own lens and make their own unique meaning from it. To be sure, meaning is always contested, is often political, and is rarely, if ever, decided by data alone—no matter how convincing we, public health professionals, believe the data to be. Because the meaning we make varies dramatically from person to person and between groups, the actions we believe are necessary vary as well. As author Anaïs Nin is frequently quoted as saying, "We don't see things as they are, we see them as *we* are." Nelson Mandela is also credited with expressing this same sentiment in his famous quote, "Where you stand depends upon where you sit."

THE IMPORTANCE OF POSITIONALITY

The considerations in the previous section point to the importance of positionality, a simple but important concept that Mandela summed up nicely. As public health professionals, we are often inclined to start with the data. We should instead start with careful self-reflection on our positionality in relation to the data and the public health topic we are considering. Starting with this will help us to better understand the impact of history, culture, and context on our life and work and will likely reveal ways in which our positionality might influence our perspectives and behaviors. For example, an epidemiologist who has personally experienced a preterm birth may be inclined to routinely examine prematurity data in her epidemiological analyses. Similarly, a public health professional of Vietnamese ancestry may consistently create Asian subpopulation options on community surveys, thereby collecting important demographic data their peers often overlook. These examples demonstrate how positionality consistently impacts how we collect, use, and interpret data.

Consider another real-life example. The authors were previously involved in a collaborative research project that explored the emotional labor of doing public health equity work.[1] We were all studying the same issue, but as we shared our personal motivations for conducting the analysis (part of our positionality), we discovered that some team members were naturally inclined to accurately measure and record the difficulty of equity work while others were driven to record and share stories. We discussed this and ultimately made the decision to embrace both perspectives. In other words, our positionality impacted our research methods, expanding the type of data we collected to include both quantitative (numeric data) and qualitative (non-numeric data assessing qualities, characteristics, and perceptions). The end result was a richer and more complete analysis.

The example in the previous paragraph demonstrates why it is critical that we attend to the positionality of others who partner with us in whatever public health challenge we are addressing. As individuals, our culture, beliefs, value systems, and moral stances shape our ways of being, knowing, and doing. Naturally, these key features that define who we are differ markedly from one person to the next. As such, when we practice self-reflection and turn our attention to the self-reflection of others, we are attending to the rich context of public health practice. The bottom line is this: our positionalities are part of the data. Rather than seeking to remove the personal element or claim complete objectivity, we often collect more data and use it more wisely when we embrace the personal. Positionality is key data in public health that should not be overlooked.

Author Positionality Statements

In this section, we provide the authors' positionality statements so readers can gain a better understanding of how we approach the use of data in public health. You will notice that the content and styles of our positionality statements differ. As authors, we did not strive for uniformity or even consistency in the structure of our positionality statements. This is because we believe in the value of our individual uniqueness and prefer to find our common ground by appreciating the diverse perspectives of others. This is true even when the unique traits of others do not merge neatly with our own, as we discovered during this writing process.

Data as Guardrails (Chad Abresch)

As a young child, my family routinely visited the Rocky Mountains for our summer vacations. My father, who was a career railroader, seemed to love the drives more than any of our destinations. His favorite drive was the Million Dollar Highway between Silverton and Ouray, Colorado. This 25-mile stretch of road cuts through steep mountain passes and takes hairpin turns around solid rock cliff faces. In most stretches, the narrow, two-lane road has no shoulders or guardrails of any kind. Just inches from your tires, the mountain plunges out of view, dropping hundreds of feet in free fall. The breathtaking scenery around every bend beckons the driver to take their eyes off the road to steal a quick glance—the views are irresistible.

On these drives, my mother vacillated between pointing out the vistas to my brother and me and grasping my father's arm as we navigated tight turns. I remember thinking how much easier it would be for my dad to drive if she wasn't holding onto him and how hard it must be for him to ignore all the beauty. But my mom insisted, "Don't look, Marvin," and he happily obliged, driving on in silence and smiling the whole time. The only words I remember him speaking were in response to my mother's repeated insistence that, "They really should install guardrails along this entire route. Wouldn't that be safer?" He would simply reply, "Sure would."

In much the same way, I view data as guardrails, helping me and others understand the parameters of various health challenges and avoid veering off in misguided directions. Like my mother's insistence, data should be present along the entire route, reminding us of who is in the car with us and providing a sense of reassurance that the actions we are taking to protect and promote the public's health are on track and moving us in the right direction.

My positionality as a public health professional emphasizes the necessity of data and is illustrated in the allegory of the guardrail. Guardrails, however, do not dictate a precise route. They are not like train tracks that predetermine the course of a locomotive. Instead, they provide parameters and some safety, giving navigators a sure sense that they are headed in the right direction—along with the confidence gained from not careening off the side of a mountain.

Understanding the limitations of data is key. Without question, data should not act as our only guide. Imagine the sparks that would fly from a vehicle hugging the guardrails throughout the entire drive. The other motorists along the route would stare in disbelief. Obviously, this would never happen. And yet, as public health professionals, we are, at times, inclined to make this very mistake. This aspect of my positionality reminds me that a singular reliance on data—data as deterministic—is peculiar and even dangerous. To counteract this tendency, we must involve our cognitive abilities to sense, think, reason, and evaluate. We must also engage community members in our work and proceed with understanding and empathy, adjusting our personal perspectives in response to the social needs and context. Indeed, the will of community members who are most impacted by the health challenges we are addressing should be preeminent in our public health decision making. Together, we examine the data, consider possible approaches, and implement and refine our strategies.

As my father navigated the tight mountain turns, consistently heeded the cautions of my mother, and even pulled off occasionally so my brother and I could check out one of the scenic overlooks, he was unknowingly providing me a perfect example of a public health professional. Humble, attentive to the voice of others, and practiced in proving safe passage for all. I'm sure he was also happy to be away from trains for a week or two.

Living Data (Regina Idoate)

I am an enrolled member of the Cherokee Nation of Oklahoma and an Associate Professor of Health Promotion, Director of Spirituality, Culture and Health, and Co-Director of Community Engagement and Outreach in the College of Public Health at the University of Nebraska Medical Center (UNMC). My previous roles include that of Division Director of Health and Wellness for the Pueblo of Tesuque and Child Development Program Evaluator for the Interdisciplinary Center for Program Evaluation at the Munroe-Meyer Institute at UNMC. I have a PhD in Preventive and Societal Medicine, master's degrees in Spanish Language and Culture and Christian Spirituality and a graduate certificate in Maternal and Child Health Epidemiology. As a social and behavioral scientist, I study community systems in relation to culture and ecology to improve population health. I have dedicated the past ten years to research, outreach, and teaching focused on advancing the health of Indigenous populations. As an Indigenous health researcher, it is my hope that everyone working with data belonging to Indigenous Peoples recognizes a sense of responsibility to work with data in ways that honor persons' relationships to the data, including those who have come before us, those who are with us now, and those who come after us. I am constantly learning how to do this better and observing the importance of decolonizing data, practicing Indigenous data sovereignty, and promoting Indigenous ways of collecting, analyzing, and disseminating data. I want my work to demonstrate the relevance of context in mobilizing communities to promote health. I believe we all have a part to play in the research process, either as researchers, participants, or audience. I believe that we are all storied beings, living datasets that are constantly growing and changing through our relationship to data. As my roles change over time, I want to have a teachable spirit. I want to collaborate across disciplines and cultures and never stop finding the time and space to play, pray, wonder, and wander.

My family, my studies, and my work have created a sense of home for me in multiple places across the United States of America and the Basque Country. I speak English and Spanish fluently and I practice both Tsalagi (Cherokee) and Euskara (Basque) daily. I am the ridiculously grateful mother to a deeply curious, joyful, creative, and empathetic Basque/Cherokee boy and auntie to three beautiful, hilarious, and strong Cherokee artists/scientists. I am the great-granddaughter of a teacher, granddaughter of an artist, and the daughter of a nurse and a builder. I am a direct descendent of Nanyehi Ward, the Beloved Cherokee woman known for being both a warrior and a peacemaker who negotiated understandings between Settlers and the Cherokee People. I stand on my ancestors' shoulders as I challenge colonized approaches to public health by working with communities to Indigenize and more importantly, localize, research and evaluation processes. As *Amatxo/Etsi* to a Basque/Cherokee child and a mentor to Indigenous youth, I work to promote healthier future generations and encourage work that respects and uplifts Indigenous peoples, families, communities, and organizations. I believe in conducting research in relational ways. I have been taught that knowledge has existed since time immemorial, and it is revealed to us through the experiences and observations we have in relationship with persons and places. To me, that means standing by the rule "nothing about us without us." In my experience, the most effective use of data involves the sovereign owners of that data in reflection, consensus building, and decision making.

Everything in the previous two paragraphs—my positionality—leads me to collect, analyze, interpret, and share data with intentionality. This is practiced through a commitment to prioritizing community values, perspectives, and protocols that aim to ensure that the data I collect and disseminate respects and uplifts the peoples, families, and communities that I have the privilege to work with. This means that I actively seek out different types of data (not only numbers and words but also art, nature, spirit, and other data) as it is relevant to the population I am working with, I collect data through community-developed measures as well as measures validated by the academy, and I work collaboratively with not only academic researchers but also community-based researchers in developing and implementing tailored data collection, analysis, interpretation, and dissemination processes. This also means that as context changes, people and processes change and data-informed decision making becomes a more iterative, ongoing practice of reflection and action that results in a continuous cycle of coming to know the data in context.

Using Data to Paint in Broad Strokes (Carol Gilbert)

Almost all the ancestors I know of had their roots in England. My grandparents on my father's side were from farm families in Massachusetts. My maternal grandmother was a social worker who came from a family of businessmen in the Philadelphia area. My maternal grandfather was an engineer who came from a family of missionaries. My parents were both college educated, as were most of my grandparents, aunts, and uncles.

My father taught at the university, and my mother stayed home, raised kids, and did volunteer work. They were Quakers (as am I). At that time, many Quakers were concerned about whether the planet could sustain the rapidly increasing human population, so after my parents had two children of their own, they adopted two boys of the Omaha people (this was before the Indian Child Welfare Act) and an African American girl. Having these siblings gave me some early glimpses of racism. My parents knew nothing about the data that showed that children of color were more likely to be removed from their homes by social services, and that this was part of a larger effort to "assimilate" Native Americans and erase their cultures.

My father and both my grandfathers were engineers, and science was clearly valued at our house. My father taught chemical engineering and liked to put on his professor's attitude when explaining things. Even when I was a child, I felt this was pretentious and patriarchal, but I see that same "colonizer" attitude in myself sometimes. My father could be genuinely humble too, and sometimes he would say, "I've already told you more than I know." He was an amateur musician. There was always music in our house, and he taught me how to play the guitar. My mother is still living and I'm lucky to be able to spend time with her. Both parents were religious and strongly ethical in the Quaker way, meaning when you know what is right you need to do it. We worked on political campaigns, attended peace marches and international students' family events, and spent one summer building a community center in a poor, Black neighborhood in Richmond, Indiana. We went to powwows, sold crafts to raise money for children in Vietnam, and always had big gardens. Our Quakerism also means there is a spiritual way of knowing, and spiritual experience counts. Having maintained connections with the Omaha culture through my brothers' families, I find much similarity between that and Quaker culture.

Now, I am a mother and a grandmother. My epidemiological priorities are doubtless influenced by the fact that two of my children have died. Our first son was a term stillbirth, and our adopted daughter died at 23 in a car crash. My husband and I are raising her son. Two of my children are grown, married, and living farther away than I would like.

My formal education included a bachelor's degree in mechanical engineering, a master's plus half a dozen additional courses in mathematical statistics, and a PhD in medical sciences interdepartmental areas, with coursework and a dissertation in public health. I've worked for CityMatCH, an agency that supports local public health departments in maternal and child health work, for two decades. Because of this work, I have past and current connections to people who care about using data to help guide public health efforts. I enjoy helping them to learn methods including interpreting and communicating their findings carefully. Part of what motivates me to include analysis of *existing data* as a first pass at understanding most situations is my aversion to wasting time and resources. It seems unethical *not* to use data that has already been collected.

I know that the mathematical assumptions required for most statistical modeling are not met in many public health contexts. For example, humans are never independent and identically distributed units. Instead, we live in families that share genes and practices. Likewise, strongly influenced by our environments, we grow to be similar to our neighbors in many ways. These circumstances make our data correlated rather than independent. Though there are methods to account for correlation, they depend on what data elements are collected, and therefore much remains unknown. This means that epidemiologists need to use robust methods, perform sensitivity analyses, and remain aware that they are painting in broad strokes. We need to interpret data findings in awareness of their limitations and always try to estimate at least in what direction we err. Many of these issues are covered in Chapters 2 and 3.

Even with its limitations, using imperfect data carefully is almost always better than relying solely on our own experience and opinions. We need the guardrails that simple facts can provide.

Honoring Place (Aislinn Rookwood)

From a demographer's viewpoint, I am a non-Hispanic White American woman. I was raised in two households, one of which was a multigenerational home that shaped my love for family, providing me with a foundational understanding of my heritage and grounding me in the importance of intergenerational connection. My family's roots come primarily from Western Europe, with my family's lineage being traced back to modern-day England and Scandinavia. My most recent connection to these roots is through my paternal grandfather, who immigrated to the Midwest from Denmark as a young adult. Our family can be traced back through him to the community of Nykøbing Falster, Denmark, near the dark waters of the Baltic Sea, where generations dwelled for hundreds of years. I have had the privilege of standing in the place of my family and feeling a profound sense of belonging that transcends words and overwhelms the senses.

As a child, I was raised in two places—one centered in a large, diverse metropolitan area in Arizona and the other in a rural community on an American Indian reservation in Montana. I was educated in Title I public schools and in spaces where White children were not viewed as a majority. I was uniquely fortunate to be educated by diverse teachers in spaces where whiteness was challenged through personal accounts and actively decentered when possible. These experiences greatly shaped my love for learning and inquiry, handing on perspectives that challenge our understanding of what we know, how we know, and why we want to know information about the world around us.

My spouse and I are transplants to a Midwestern city that is now the hometown of our two children. As a transplant to this community, it is my responsibility to educate and inform myself of the historical and present context of the place in which I live and work. This is a value I have impressed upon my children by engaging in our community through play and work. We have created a multigenerational home where we encourage them to explore and foster the development of their identities as multiracial people (White and Black/African American) and as Jamaican and American citizens. The work and education of me and my spouse has significantly changed the social mobility of our family and children.

I was considered a low-income, first-generation college student. I would not have completed my education without the support of a community college in Phoenix, Arizona, Phoenix College, where I received my associate of science in biology. Once I completed this milestone, I transferred to the Mel and Enid Zuckerman College of Public Health at the University of Arizona in Tucson, Arizona to obtain my bachelor of science in public health with a minor in soil and water science, followed by a master of public health in environmental and occupational health. I completed my PhD in health promotion and disease prevention research at UNMC in Omaha, Nebraska. The scholarship of Indigenous and Black researchers and practitioners has been foundational and transformational in my education. Outside of higher education institutions, my education has been greatly influenced by the communities I have been fortunate to work with or alongside and the places I have lived.

I currently work in the College of Public Health, where my work is focused on understanding how to better address disparities in children's environmental health. As a researcher, I believe it is my ethical and moral duty to ensure that the methodologies and results of my research reflect the lived experiences of the individuals and communities researched through community-engaged approaches. Furthermore, it is my responsibility to ensure that the research conducted is balanced with action. My aim in research is that the data we collect, request, analyze, interpret, and share as part of public health programs honors the places and spaces we represent. As you read this book, I hope that you find it a useful guide to help align your work with this aim and that it challenges you to consider the questions that we ask, how we ask them, and why we are asking them.

Data as an Identity (El Kerns)

I am a general American mutt. My ancestors at least three generations back were all born and raised in the Midwest with only the most recent generation growing up in a large metro area. Prior generations all lived in small towns in Missouri or Kansas. My best guess is that I have some mix of mostly Western European origins, but this is only a guess. I mark non-Hispanic White on forms asking my race/ethnicity because that is what others perceive me to be. I have never really felt strong ties to any particular group no matter the classifier (e.g., race, religion, social class).

I grew up experiencing many different variations of these groups depending on which parental figure(s) were involved in my life at the time. I went to a Catholic kindergarten, an elementary school on the outer edge of suburbia, an inner-city middle school, and a wealthy suburban high school. Given this ever-changing environment, I developed no allegiance to a given identity. I suppose this is why I have zero interest in sports and have a hard time understanding the appeal of nationalism. If you have no deeply ingrained pride or emotional investment in the success of a given team/group/nation, then the appeal of "winning" just isn't there. I acknowledge this as a limitation in my perspective when studying those who do have a strong sense of community as a driver of their behaviors.

A few things my childhood did instill in me were a strong drive to promote equity and a firm belief in the power of data. I witnessed firsthand how varied one's opportunities, educational quality, and access to resources can be in childhood. The impact of these circumstances on one's ability to achieve and maintain their desired quality of life was reinforced by my educational pursuits. I spent the entirety of my twenties in educational programs: first, a bachelor's degree in biology; second, a master's in public health epidemiology; third, a fellowship in epidemiology at the National Institute of Occupational Safety and Health; and finally, a PhD in biomedical informatics. Throughout, I worked full time at educational and health institutions with roles that increasingly specialized in storing, retrieving, analyzing, and presenting data. This instilled in me an appreciation for the power of data. I feel these roles and my education define who I am far better than any of the traditional ways people are usually grouped. To me, these are more important data points in the synthesis of my positionality. Not only have I leveraged data to solve the many research questions I have encountered, but my ability to find it, wrangle it, and present it in a way that others can use has given me a strong sense of my identity and value.

Currently, I have a variety of roles at both a university and a pediatric hospital, which all revolve around optimizing how these institutions leverage information systems for both operational and research purposes. In these roles, I bring together my experience and understanding of databases as well as expertise in the fields of usability and design to represent data in a trusted and understandable format for answering questions and making decisions. For example, I created a tool that clinicians could use to define inclusion criteria, exclusion criteria, and metrics of interest for care pathways they were implementing. This tool facilitates handoff to hospital report writers so both groups are on the same page as to how metrics were defined. I also created a standardized dashboard template for displaying metrics for qualifying patients that included the definitions for criteria and metrics, metric numerator and denominator values, and charted performance over time. This dashboard template allows the evaluation of pathway success to be consistent and understandable by both the clinical stakeholders and the technical personnel building the individual pathway dashboards. This process required me to incorporate my understanding of electronic health record databases, clinical stakeholder decision making process needs, data visualization, and the impact of clear definitions and standards on trust.

Data are everywhere and have incredible potential to improve the efficiency and effectiveness of health care and public health systems. Yet, most data sources are underutilized and even those used more frequently are often misrepresented. This is due to a variety of factors, including lack of access, limitations on quality, lack of adequate representation within the data source, competing interests between the data "owners" and data "users," inconsistent rules and policies, and so much more. My hope is that this book gives public health practitioners the tools to make the most of this valuable resource while accounting for its limitations.

DEVELOPING YOUR OWN POSITIONALITY STATEMENT

As discussed in the previous section, positionality statements are fundamental to the entire inquiry and data use process. They impact the types of questions we ask, the data we look at to answer questions, the analytic processes we employ, and the interpretation of findings. Now that you have read the authors' positionality statements, it's time to develop your own. Spend time working through the Positionality Exercise included in Appendix 1A. As you do, select a public health topic of importance to you and your community. Answer the questions while considering how your views are shaped not only by the available data, but also by your positionality in relation to the data.

Be careful not to skip the important work of positionality or gloss over its significance. In making our careers in public health, we have an opportunity to serve our entire community by safeguarding and improving health. This is a profound opportunity and responsibility. Becoming clear about *where we sit* is essential in developing effective public health leadership.

REFERENCES

1. Abresch C, Gilbert C, Johnson M, et al. Understanding the emotional labor of public health equity work: A mixed methods study. *J Racial Ethn Health Disparities*. 2023;10(3):1047–1057. doi:10.1007/s40615-022-01292-9

Appendix 1A: Positionality Exercise—Writing Your Positionality Statement

WHAT IS A POSITIONALITY STATEMENT?

A positionality statement is a written or oral declaration of awareness of your own socially constructed position in society and the role that your position plays in the production of knowledge. It is important for us to consider positionality because it strongly impacts how we collect, use, and interpret data. This is a testament to what you know and what you can and perhaps cannot know. There are three steps to establish your positionality: (1) locate yourself in relation to the purpose and meaning of the project you are working on; (2) locate yourself in relation to everyone involved in the project; and (3) locate yourself in relation to the context and process of the project.[1]

WHY DOES POSITIONALITY MATTER?

Our practices and presumptions are fundamentally shaped by the values that underpin our concept of self and of others. Our perspectives about how the world operates and our place within it shape key actions we take in life. And our understanding about how knowledge is construed, and who the knowers are, often determines how we go about making important decisions in life. No person, regardless of their role, can be purely objective. Whether an artist or subject, health professional or patient, student or teacher, researcher or participant, evaluator or end user, funder or grantee, you filter what you see through the experiences you have had. Your lens, background, and position will affect what you choose to explore, the exact questions you ask, the population you choose to work with, the angle of your investigation, the methods judged most adequate for engaging in that process, your interpretation of findings, and your framing and communication of conclusions.[2] It is an ethical duty to intentionally and mindfully attend to your roles in this process by establishing your positionality at the outset of every project and to engage continuously in reflexivity throughout the process. By questioning, critically reflecting on, and stating your positionality, you can strengthen the validity of your methods and safeguard the ethics of the process.

STEP 1: SELF-REFLECTION

Consider the following list of self-reflexive questions. For each section, write short responses to the questions. Allow your energy to guide your effort. For questions where you have a lot to write, let your responses flow. Conversely, on questions where little seems to come to mind, do not feel obligated to force your response.

Once you have completed each section, consider your responses. Here is the time to ask why you had more to write on some questions than others. Is there something significant in that which merits more consideration?

Where Are You From?

- What is your heritage?
- Who are your ancestors?
- What ways of knowing, being, and doing have been passed down to you?
- What is the history of the places and peoples you belong to?
- Do you have any existing connections with the population participating in the project? If so, in what ways?
- Do you have any existing connections with the subject matter of focus in the project? If so, in what ways?
- Does this project challenge your positionality in any way?

Where Have You Been?

- What places have you called home?
- What life events have greatly affected you?
- How would you describe your background?
- How have you changed over time?
- What mediums, measures, and methods do you have experience using?
- Do you have any lived experiences that influence your perspective or approach on the public health topic you are currently addressing? If so, in what ways?
- Do you have any lived experiences that influence your interest in or approach to the population you are working with? If so, in what ways?

Where Are You Now?

- How do you self-identify? What is your biological sex and gender identity? Your age group? Your social class? Your vocation?
- What are your beliefs, values, and religious and political orientations?

- What stereotypes do you hold?
- Which factors about your current work and projects are most significant to you?
- What are your preferred ways of knowing? Being? Doing?
- What are your beliefs about the topic of this project?
- What are your beliefs about the population participating in this project?
- Do your identity, context, lived experience, and worldview align with or conflict with the design and process of your current projects? If so, in what ways?
- What is your understanding of systems of oppression that may be at work in your current projects? What is their influence on you and others in this work?

Where Are You Going?

- What are your goals related to your work?
- How do you envision your current projects going?
- What results do you think you will find in your projects?
- What is your vision of equity in relation to your projects?
- What are your hopes for your projects?
- What are your hopes for the people participating in your projects?
- What would you like to contribute to the field through your work?

How Do You Define Data and What Does That Mean to You?

- How do you define data?
- Is your response to the previous question indicative of a broad definition of data that encompasses qualitative as well as quantitative information? Does it include art and other forms of cultural expression? Or do you view data as strictly numeric and believe it is important to have distinctions between numbers, stories, and art?
- What role do you think data should play in public health decision making? Do you believe it is a starting point for conversations with affected communities or should it be given more weight?

STEP 2: DRAFT YOUR POSITIONALITY STATEMENT

Once you have completed the questions in Step 1, begin drafting your positionality statement. This is your statement, so remember that you make the rules. You are not bound by the questions in this exercise and should not feel obligated to shape a statement that is a collection of section-by-section responses. Instead, write what comes. Write about who you are, knowing you have done the work to inform that process by considering each of the questions in Step 1.

STEP 3: SHARE WITH OTHERS

Positionality statements are deeply personal. They are also meant to be shared. When we share our positionality, others come to know what matters most to us and what drives our passions and actions in the work we do.

If you have never developed or shared your positionality statement before, consider starting with a close and trusted colleague. Or perhaps even a family member. Once you build confidence in sharing your statement, you can become more open with others, even encouraging them to take on this critical self-reflexive work themselves.

STEP 4: ATTEND TO YOUR POSITIONALITY (AND THE POSITIONALITY OF OTHERS)

Unfortunately, the hard work of developing a positionality statement can be forgotten all too quickly. This happens especially easily when we are working on complex, challenging, or contentious projects. In these intense moments, our emotions can take over and later we are likely to find ourselves thinking, "I certainly could have handled that situation better."

To counteract this common human tendency, make sure to revisit your positionality statement frequently. Try to predict potentially challenging meetings or interactions and remind yourself of your positionality prior to these events. Another effective strategy is to intentionally shape meeting agendas to include positionality work. During long planning sessions or retreats, this may involve using the positionality exercise here, but shorter exercises and icebreakers can be designed to draw in certain key questions from the list in Step 1. These questions will help situate all participants in our individual uniqueness while reminding us that we also share much in common.

REFERENCES

1. Savin-Baden M, Major C. *Qualitative Research: The Essential Guide to Theory and Practice.* Routledge; 2023.
2. Malterud K. Qualitative research: Standards, challenges, and guidelines. *Lancet.* 2001;358 (9280):483–488. doi:10.1016/S0140-6736(01)05627-6

2

Data for Public Health Practice

Public health practice relies on many types of evidence, and scientific literature may be the most important of these. However, our evidence must also include epidemiological and in-depth qualitative knowledge about the communities we are working with and aiming to serve. For example, research has shown that the prone infant sleep position is an important contributor to sleep-related infant death (SIDS and SUID), but only local data can tell us whether people in our community are using the prone position. In some places, we find that parents are using the prone infant sleep position by putting babies to sleep on their backs, but the real issue may be other behaviors such as co-sleeping and use of pillows or blankets. For good decision making, we also need to understand local cultural beliefs and environmental conditions that influence parental behavior. A simple educational message may not be effective if there is a cultural belief that co-sleeping is healthiest or if parents are dealing with cold temperatures or vermin in the house. When we are not informed of such community factors, our public health campaigns miss the mark. Even if public health practitioners live in the community of interest and stay informed about the local program and policy landscape, public health decisions will require local population-based data and ongoing involvement of community members across all relevant sectors of society. Both qualitative reviews and statistical summaries that describe health outcomes and risk factors can help identify important issues and help prioritize resources. Resource priorities that might emerge could include time and money for more in-depth investigations to inform design and implementation of program and policy changes.

Good decision making requires extensive contextual information, including knowledge of the community's resources, leadership, existing efforts, needs, mores, and subcultures. Maintaining enduring relationships with the people served helps make contextual information available and helps assure that the right interventions are chosen or designed and implemented successfully.[1] Good models for such relationships are multisector collaboratives formed around a given health or health determinant topic such as Generate Health in St. Louis, Missouri.[2] In this countywide public–private collaborative, a diverse set of partners from dozens of sectors came together, initially to establish priorities that centered on improving health care access and utilization to improve the health of women, children, and families. The collaborative remains active nearly a quarter century after its founding and includes a data hub, which is still used to establish new priorities and areas for action.

The Fetal Infant Mortality Review (FIMR) is a second example that involves multisector partners in both data collection and decision making.[3] In FIMR, a multisector committee from the community conducts detailed reviews of fetal and infant deaths to identify patterns and system problems that are then addressed by a second community committee.[4] Because of the FIMR model's success in addressing fetal and infant mortality, it has been adapted to address other salient health concerns. For example, CityMatCH—a national organization representing maternal and child health programs in urban public health departments—in collaboration with the Centers for Disease Control and Prevention (CDC), adapted FIMR to enable states and communities to review cases of perinatal HIV exposure. The adapted model was effective in using data to identify where gaps in care were resulting in the vertical transmission of HIV. Through careful review and action, these gaps could be closed, resulting in fewer cases of transmission. Combined with other important prevention efforts, this work contributed to the national elimination of perinatal HIV. Today, the FIMR model is being adapted to address additional issues, including maternal morbidity and mortality and congenital syphilis.

SCIENTIFIC LITERATURE

To develop a basic understanding of a public health issue's contributing factors, effective interventions, and commonly used data sources and measures, we recommend beginning by seeking out literature reviews and existing databases on "what works." Much scientific literature is available to the public from PubMed (https://pubmed.ncbi.nlm.nih.gov) and from organizations that produce high-quality literature reviews, including the Cochrane Collaboration,[5] The Campbell Collaboration,[6] the Agency for Healthcare Research and Quality (AHRQ),[7] The Centre for Reviews and Dissemination,[8] and the Community Guide.[9] Though many documents are free and can be easily found online through Google Scholar or publishers such as those mentioned here, accessing some scientific literature databases can be expensive. If you do not have access to online literature databases through your agency, we recommend working with local universities and public libraries to gain access through guest user accounts or partnerships.

In addition to rigorous reviews, practitioners should consider seeking out literature by researchers with diverse perspectives and "white papers" from governmental and nongovernmental organizations. Reading original sources, rather than relying on media reports of study results and AI-generated summaries, will allow you to better assess the quality of the evidence and diversity of perspectives. Take time to understand the context and populations that have been studied and consider whether they apply to your population. One issue to be aware of when making use of the scientific literature is the potential for misinformation coming from preprints. Scientific manuscripts undergo intense scrutiny from multiple other scientists prior to publication. This peer review process is typically double blinded—the authors do not know the reviewers and vice versa. The review process is slow, sometimes painfully so, but it greatly helps to ensure quality and accuracy. Preprints allow scientists to publish their work immediately, often while the review process is ongoing. They are also freely available to everyone and, therefore, often get substantial media attention. In this way, preprints allow for the faster dissemination of new knowledge, but without undergoing the scrutiny of other scientists in the field, their findings can be erroneous. Public health practitioners need to exercise great caution when basing decisions about the public's health on unreviewed preprints. In most instances, it will be better to watch these articles and their findings closely to see how they emerge after review.

When high-quality literature reviews are not available for your specific topic or not applicable to your population or circumstances, you can critically appraise individual published studies or even conduct a literature review yourself. The detailed review criteria and processes published on the websites of organizations like Cochrane and AHRQ can serve as guides for those who want to assess the quality of evidence from any study. Other extremely valuable resources include databases of curated, evidence-based practices that address particular outcomes and indicate the level of evidence that supports the practice's effectiveness. Examples of these are County Health Rankings & Roadmaps and The MCH Evidence Center. The Community Tool Box maintains a list of databases of best practices for various public health fields (https://ctb.ku.edu/en/databases-best-practices). An important feature of many of these databases is the inclusion of practices that are emerging or have little supporting evidence, and even practices that have evidence against them. The MCH Evidence Center includes practices for which the main existing evidence is "expert opinion." This feature is important because of limitations of the published scientific literature, outlined in the following paragraphs.

Each source of information for decision making has limitations, and scientific evidence is no exception. The most obvious limitation may be lack of evidence on many topics of interest to health departments. Original studies can take years to obtain funding for, carry out, and publish. Research that is based on secondary analysis of existing data sources can only be as up-to-date as the sources are. Further weaknesses may not be as obvious. The research pipeline is affected by biases of funding sources, including governments, foundations, and commercial funders.[10] There are many ways to bias study design and analytic methods once projects are funded (discussed in Chapter 3),[11] and additional biases affect whether studies get published or not.[12] We conclude that, because of the urgency of our communities' needs and the limitations of scientific information, public health must sometimes "go out on a limb" and implement unproven interventions. Nevertheless, it is important that we are both internally aware and transparent with the public when we are making these decisions to ensure that we build evidence rather than magnifying errors.

Last, before selecting an "evidence-based" or "evidence-informed" policy or practice, verify that it is described thoroughly enough that you can adopt it with fidelity or adapt it to your context. Often, the authors or the agencies that implemented the program can be contacted for details, but documentation is a common shortcoming in public health practice. As your health department works to implement programs or policies, keep in mind that you are producing evidence, and if you carefully document your work, it can become part of the evidence base that other health departments can build from.

SECONDARY DATA

Secondary data are data that have previously been collected and are available for analysis. There are many sources of secondary data that cover a large array of public health topics and reach the national, state, and local levels. While you didn't collect these data yourself, they are a rich source of information about a community's health and potential challenges. One of the important ways to learn about a community's health issues is by using local data from sources that already exist. Broad categories of secondary data include administrative data (collected as part of routine operations of a given organization), survey data (collected with the intent to answer specific questions), case reports, surveillance systems, registries, and place-based data. CDC provides an excellent and well-maintained inventory of important public health secondary data sources on their website.[13] Another excellent source for these data is data.gov.[14]

It is important to determine whether the data source you are planning to use is population-based and if so, what "population" it represents. Population-based data sources are designed either to include or to represent everyone in the population of interest, with methodologies that vary depending on the topic. Many sources of population-based data contain information about individuals that can be summarized at the levels of the nation, states, counties, or even smaller areas. Examples include administrative data sources like the Decennial Census and Birth Certificate Vital Records Data (which do include nearly everyone); representative sample surveys such as the American Community Survey; the Pregnancy Risk Assessment Monitoring System (PRAMS) that represents the population of all pregnancies resulting in a live birth; the Behavior Risk Factor Surveillance System (BRFSS) that represents people aged 18 and older; and the Youth Risk Behavior Surveillance System (YRBSS) that represents high school students. Generally, nationally representative research datasets such as the National Longitudinal Mortality Survey or the National Survey of Family Growth cannot be used to learn about states and counties because they are not designed to include enough people for stable estimates, or locations are not identified, or appropriate statistical weights are not available.

To be useful for public health, each data source must provide documentation, including a codebook that explains the variables and the values represented by the codes. At a minimum, the analyst must become intimately familiar with the codebook, never assuming what a variable or value means based on its name. The analyst should delve deeply into the documentation to learn how to use the dataset, including the standard measures it produces, its limitations, and its methods for data collection, statistical modeling, and weighting.

For survey data, another important consideration is weighting. Weighting is a process that can be used for survey data sources to account for the fact that response rates are not random but vary by respondent characteristics. Weighting is not required for datasets that include the whole population of interest. However, for most samples, the distribution of the dataset does not match the distribution of the whole population, and weights must be constructed to produce unbiased estimates. Examples of weighted datasets include the National Health and Nutrition Examination Survey and BRFSS, both of which include multiple weighting variables for different types of analyses. Conversely, the nation's vital records system provides datasets that are unweighted, as they include entire populations. If response rates varied based on just one factor, such as age, it would be easy to create appropriate weights. For example, if teens were half as likely to respond as others, each teen respondent would receive a weight of 2 and be "counted" twice in the analysis. Actual weights are constructed based on many factors and using several methods, often in combination.[15] Weighting variables included in the dataset tell the analysis software how many cases each survey response should "count" for to make survey results represent the whole population. Different sets of weights may be included in the dataset to allow analyses to represent different whole populations. For example, one weighting variable should be used if the analysis is to represent the state, and another if it is to represent counties. The accuracy of weights varies, and analysts can seek out validation studies[16] or verify accuracy themselves based on whole-population summary data if it is available. Using the data without weights would create results that represent only the individuals included in the dataset, skewing results towards the characteristics of subpopulations who were oversampled.

Public health professionals can also make use of disease surveillance systems and registries, even though they are generally not population based. Surveillance systems such as the National Respiratory and Enteric Virus Surveillance System track the incidence and prevalence of various diseases and conditions within populations. These are often maintained nationally by CDC. Registries that track cases of specific diseases or conditions[17,18] can be government run or maintained by professional societies with an interest in the given disease (e.g., the Society of Thoracic Surgeons runs the national registry for heart surgeries). Registries with mandated reporting, such as many maintained by CDC,[19] have the great advantage of being more complete than those with voluntary reporting, such as those maintained by professional or academic groups. A database of CDC-reportable diseases is available through a query system found on CDC WONDER.[20] However, diseases must usually be diagnosed by a physician to be reported, so diseases with mild symptoms in some patients tend to be underreported.

Health care and health outcome data are also available through administrative databases created from insurance claims or provider billing data. These contain information on patients' encounters with health care providers, including diagnosis and procedure codes that billing is based on. The representativeness of billing data depends on inclusion rules. For example, Medicaid data includes information about health care services and pharmaceuticals for all currently enrolled patients, with enrollment changing from month to month. Medicaid enrollees meet low-income or disability requirements that vary by state. Medicare claims include data from patients aged 65 and older and patients with certain disabling diseases. Not all people aged 65 and older are enrolled, and not all enrolled people receive health care in a given time period. Several states and some private companies maintain all-payer claims databases,[21] which include claims from Medicare, Medicaid, and (ostensibly) all other insurers. The Pediatric Health Information System[22] includes data from participating freestanding children's hospitals regardless of payer (insurer), but children seen at other types of hospitals are not included.

Another important administrative data source that is available to varying degrees for public health use is Electronic Health Record (EHR) data, which is patient data collected by health care providers. EHR databases include health information such as lab results and records of encounters, diagnoses, and procedures. Some health care systems across the country have opted to participate in one of the national common data models (CDMs).[23] These health systems have normalized their EHR data to standard terminologies, rearranged it to fit the selected CDM, and have agreed to make it available for projects with approved applications. Normalized EHR data are often assembled into coordinated Health Information Exchanges (HIEs) to facilitate care across institutions. Some states have very robust HIEs, which include records about individual patient encounters from *all* health institutions in the state,[24] while other states have multiple standalone HIEs. However, even the more robust HIEs are limited to representing individuals who have received health care, and much of the data has not been standardized to the degree outlined by the CDMs.

Another important category of existing data that can be used for public health work is geo-location or place-based data. For these databases, an individual is not the unit of analysis; instead, the individual records are *places* such as states, counties, cities, hospitals, or census tracts. Place-based databases contain information about the *place*, including the environment, the economy, crime, and other factors. They can also include averages of data from the many individuals who live there. Sources of place-based data that summarize the individuals living there should provide detailed documentation of the data source(s), years collected, and construction of measures (such as numerator and denominator). The methodology and sources section on the County Health Rankings & Roadmaps website is a good example of appropriate documentation.[25] These datasets can be *linked* to datasets about individuals that have a location variable. Linkage allows, for example, estimation of the impact of place-based factors on individual health risk behaviors or outcomes. Of course, the most useful level of place-based data is the exact address. While this is available to public health professionals in some locations within administrative data sources like birth and death certificates, it is not available for most place-based data sources, particularly those that are accessible and contain information about individuals, because this is a very risky identifier.

Many publicly available, place-based datasets can be found online. Nearly 300,000 government-run geo-datasets are currently indexed on the data.gov website.[14] Place-based summary data on certain health outcomes, socioeconomic factors, and health care resources can be found on websites such as CDC WONDER,[16] CDC PLACES,[26] the US Census Bureau's Small Area Income and Poverty Estimates Program,[27] IPUMS[28] for Census Bureau data, diversitydatakids.org,[29] the Health Resources and Services Administration's Area Health Resource Files,[30] Youth Online (for YRBSS),[25] the Kids Count Data Center,[31] and the County Health Rankings & Roadmaps.[32] CDC maintains a webpage of data sources that provide community-level information in their Public Health Professionals Gateway.[33]

It is also possible to purchase place-based marketing data for public health use from private companies such as Nielsen, which collects media utilization data, and International Data Group, which collects consumer purchasing data. Some geo-datasets are available online with the purchase of software such as ArcGIS and Tableau. When utilizing these datasets, it is important to critically review the original data sources and cite these sources appropriately. In the case of ArcGIS Online, any user can create and publish datasets, which means that some datasets could be inaccurate. We recommend utilizing datasets created by government agencies.

Many community organization and study-based datasets exist and can be found in topic-based data repositories.[34] Study-based data resources are growing exponentially due to a new National Institutes of Health rule requiring all funded studies to contribute their data to one of these repositories.

SECONDARY DATA: ADVANTAGES AND DISADVANTAGES

Public health practice can benefit from the routine use of relevant secondary data sources like those listed in the previous section. When used carefully, they produce results that serve as guardrails for our decision making process. The fact that they already exist is a big advantage. Their collection processes and contents are documented. Often, their validity has been studied and tested. Many measures in common use are based on these sources, which means we can easily compare our community with published results from other communities. Some are publicly available at no cost; others are available to health departments because they have a statutory responsibility to monitor health and risk factors. Usually, the cost is only the time required to learn their contents, idiosyncrasies, and methods for use, and the time required to carry out analyses.

However, secondary data sources have inherent limitations that can make our guardrails useless or even harmful if users don't take the time to understand and account for them. The first limitation was mentioned previously: many of these sources include only parts of the population, and these subpopulations might not represent the population we need to study the issue at hand. For example, YRBSS data are not suitable for studying children who aren't attending high school, and hospital discharge data would not help us understand diseases that don't require hospitalization.

Second, because each data source was set up for a specific purpose, these sources include only the limited information needed to fulfill those purposes. Even when the purpose of a data source is closely related to the topic at hand, such as state and regional cancer registries or BRFSS for heart disease, its scope will have inherent limitations and may not identify specific subpopulations of interest (such as neighborhood, race, or tribal affiliation). The weighting of sample datasets is not perfect, as mentioned in the previous section, and ostensibly even whole-population datasets may have coverage problems. Some examples of population datasets with known coverage gaps include vital records whose infant death files are known to underreport very low-birth-weight deaths in some states[35] and the Decennial Census, which underreports young children.[36]

A further caution to be aware of when using secondary data sources is that they were not intentionally designed to capture the specific motives, support systems, or cultural differences that could be important to determine whether a proposed or current intervention will succeed or fail. Further, because the data were collected sometime in the past, the ability of study designs using only secondary data to determine cause-and-effect relationships is necessarily limited. Sole reliance on secondary data can limit our thinking because we only have variables that someone else has already decided are important.

Another notable limitation of quantitative secondary data is the problem of small numbers. For both statistical validity and privacy reasons, small geographical areas and groups with small population sizes are often not represented in studies and reports. This is more often an issue in secondary data because the identity variable of interest may not be collected, and because (in surveys) the group may not be oversampled as it would need to be for inclusion in a study. This results in erasure: the systematic ignoring of some groups and loss of the granularity needed to understand the true underlying variation in outcomes. Finally, few secondary datasets were designed by members of the populations that public health serves, such as parents of toddlers, people with HIV, or people who are unemployed. While the design of surveys and studies requires extensive training to yield reliable results, the routine input of community members and affected populations would improve data collection instruments, producing more usable and accurate findings.

PRIMARY DATA

We can address some of the limitations of secondary data sources through careful analysis and interpretation, but even if data collection processes were perfect, all questions were answered truthfully and without errors, and analyses were appropriate and unbiased, secondary data sources often do not provide all the answers we need for good decision making. Sometimes this means that we need to collect our own data, which is referred to as primary data.

Methods for primary data collection are very broad and may include surveys and interviews, often with open-ended questions, focus groups, observation of environments and activities, or even using art to elicit ideas. Like secondary data, primary data can be either quantitative (numeric data) or qualitative (non-numeric data assessing qualities, characteristics, and perceptions). Qualitative research methods allow us to collect descriptive information that is observed and described rather than measured or counted. Qualitative data can be in the form of text, symbols, audio, video, and photographs. Fine points such as colors, textures, smells, tastes, appearance, aesthetics, thoughts, feelings, opinions, emotions, and sensations help establish context and gain an in-depth understanding of the topic. For those who are new to qualitative data collection, the *CDC Field Epidemiology Manual*[37] offers an overview and guidance for qualitative data collection for public health.

It is important to note that, like quantitative data collection and analysis, collecting and analyzing qualitative data is demanding, requiring extensive training and the use of exacting methodological processes.

An exemplar of primary data collection is the Fetal Infant Mortality Review (FIMR) process described in this chapter's introduction.[4] In its full implementation, FIMR utilizes both secondary and primary data. Secondary data are gathered and summarized from existing medical charts. Primary data are collected through in-home interviews with the parents who suffered the fetal or infant loss. Ideally, FIMR teams also consider scientific literature and local population-based data.[38] Once collected, all data are shared with a local, multidisciplinary case review team to garner broad community input and expertise. In this way, FIMR is a system for continually collecting all types of data—secondary and primary, quantitative and qualitative—and using those data to engage the community to make data-informed decisions for public health improvements.

PRIMARY DATA: ADVANTAGES AND DISADVANTAGES

In addition to the opportunity to collect the precise information your project needs, primary data collection also offers opportunities for collaboration and community involvement in all phases of project development, including design, data collection, analysis, and interpretation. Another advantage of primary data collection, specifically qualitative primary data collection, is the ability to ask open-ended questions to elicit ideas that we would not have previously considered. This type of qualitative data collection is often referred to as exploratory. Exploratory data collection is important for the generation of new hypotheses and theories.

A final advantage of primary data collection that is worth noting is the enhanced ability to determine cause-and-effect relationships. While it is possible to assess causality using secondary data, the most straightforward approach is through careful study design and implementation of a primary data collection methodology. This helps to ensure that the correct and exact variables are collected from the precise population of interest in the intended time sequence. In other words, it allows for the maximum number of limitations to be intentionally designed out of the data.

The most obvious disadvantages of primary data collection include the time and expense required to collect the data. Additionally, collecting primary data places a burden on the data providers, who must respond to our surveys or sit down with us for interviews. While this can be a welcome burden, it can also be time consuming and even emotionally burdensome when the data being collected deal with difficult issues such as disease and death within their family or community. A less obvious disadvantage of primary data collection is the fact that it is difficult (often impossible) to obtain a complete list of the population you want to learn about. Such a list, sometimes called a sampling frame, allows investigators to select a representative sample. This is important in quantitative data collection efforts that seek to produce results that are generalizable for an entire population—something researchers refer to as a representative sample. In the absence of a sampling frame, many data collection efforts use convenience samples of various types, including snowball sampling (e.g., asking people on a list to recruit people they know).[39] Though more formal link-tracing methods[40] offer ways to improve the representativeness of samples selected in this way, these methods generally do not produce representative data and can inadvertently exclude hard-to-reach people, along with their experiences and ideas. If we don't have a list of the whole population of interest, we can't assess whether our sample is representative or not.

A further disadvantage of primary data collection is that when we design our own data collection methods and instruments, we often have limited opportunity to test, debug, and validate them, so our limitations are usually not known until after data collection is complete. Before developing a novel primary data collection method, it is important to review what validated instruments exist in the research and programmatic literature. Using existing instruments can mitigate some of the disadvantages regarding validation that were discussed in previous paragraphs. Conducting a thorough review of the literature is critical to ensuring the relevancy and reproducibility of your findings. Some examples of instruments that could be relevant to your programmatic work are quality-of-life measures, screening surveys, and satisfaction surveys (i.e., doctor grades). Many of these instruments are required by the Center for Medicaid Services or are utilized in clinical care. If you are unsure what instruments may be utilized in clinical care, contacting local health care organizations may be an appropriate strategy for identifying these instruments.

As we noted, the design of even a simple primary data collection instrument is complex, and when we use this approach, we must recognize that we ourselves have perspectives, assumptions, and values that affect design elements such as word choice and the structure of questions. One recommended technique for designing primary data collection instruments is to draft the story you expect to tell based on your future data, including a background section, methods, an array of possible results, and a conclusion. This technique helps you understand which questions you need versus which would merely be interesting. Unneeded questions burden your respondents and lower participation rates. An additional indispensable technique is to pilot your primary data collection instrument with a few people from your intended population, preferably people from a variety of backgrounds. Reviewing pilot data can help to tell you whether your instrument is capturing the intended data accurately. Conversations with pilot participants can help you identify and either modify or omit data collection efforts that are ambiguous, confusing, sensitive, difficult to answer, or even offensive. Language that is perceived as racist, sexist, or politically biased can alienate potential respondents and bias your findings by not equally representing certain segments of your population.

The menu of choices you allow your respondents to select from can also bias your results. A great example of this comes from the PRAMS national survey. For more than a decade, the PRAMS survey assessed pregnancy intendedness by asking whether the person had wanted to become pregnant "then" or "sooner," interpreting these answers as "intended," versus "later" or "never," interpreting these answers as "unintended." After a fifth category ("I wasn't sure what I wanted") was added, the percentages of people choosing the two "unintended" options decreased substantially. Apparently, many people who reported an unintended pregnancy in the earlier version of the survey were unsure what they wanted, but the survey had not allowed them to select that option.[41]

Primary data collection can be improved by taking advantage of software that can check for unlikely values and common errors (e.g., Likert scale reversals) and can validate respondents' street addresses by geo-coding them when the data are being entered. Finally, always remember that primary data collection methods should be carefully documented to reduce misinterpretation by future data users and to facilitate publication.

THE IMPORTANCE OF BIAS

Whether we use data sources that already exist or collect our own data, we need to be aware of characteristics that could lead to biased measures, conclusions, or decisions. Biased measures are estimates that are different enough from the "true" value to lead to wrong decisions. Bias that leads to untruth can enter a study long before statistics are calculated. It can be introduced because of the motivation for doing the study, the perspective of the sponsors and the people designing the data collection instruments, or because of institutionalized practices or traditions. Bias can be introduced because of who is included in the dataset, the wording of questions, who provides the information, what data elements it contains, the assumptions behind how populations are grouped, and the values implicit in the analytic model we choose. Finally, bias can be caused by how we communicate the findings and how findings influence decisions.

We illustrate the impact of simple measurement bias using the case of an uncalibrated hospital scale. Of course, if a hospital weighs newborns using a scale that consistently reads half a pound low, our recorded birth weights will all be incorrect. Furthermore, our hospital's *measure* of low-birth-weight percentage will be larger than our hospital's true low-birth-weight percentage. If we can only see birth weight through the biased lens provided by this newborn scale, the problem will be difficult to gauge accurately. It is likely that we will continue to produce biased results until we calibrate the scale. This could lead to poor decisions such as misallocation of resources. If the local public health agency notices that our hospital has a higher low-birth-weight percentage than other hospitals, the epidemiologists might investigate this apparent health disparity. If they begin by questioning the data quality, they will likely find the true problem quickly. Otherwise, it's likely that more resources will be expended investigating health disparities, and it's possible that programmatic resources could be diverted unnecessarily to address a low-birth-weight problem that doesn't exist.

SOURCES OF BIAS

One potential cause of biased findings is differences in survey response rates (i.e., differential reporting). In general, to be useful for decision making (for surveillance, risk assessment, or program/policy evaluation), data sources should have consistency across person, place, and time. This is because analyses use comparisons to make numbers meaningful. A single statistic, such as a Black infant mortality rate of 7.5 in your county, is not meaningful until it is compared with another group (person), another place (state or nation), or another time (previous years). If we know that the White infant mortality rate in the same jurisdiction is 4.5, or that the corresponding state rate is 8.5, or that the Black infant mortality rate has been decreasing for the past five years, we can interpret that statistic in actionable terms. If data are not collected and processed with consistency across person, place, and time, our comparisons can be biased, and our conclusions can be wrong.

Ideally, we draw a random sample from a list (a sampling frame) that includes the entire population of interest. Because there isn't a comprehensive list of people living in a typical jurisdiction or in the United States as a whole, the American Community Survey uses a list of addresses.[42] BRFSS and other health surveys use random digit dialing to interview people on cell phones and landlines, YRBSS uses lists of schools and classes,[43] and administrative datasets use lists of enrollees or patients. Vital records data are (nearly) complete lists of people, but only at two points in time (at most): at birth and at death. These data collection systems exist for specific purposes, and their inclusion criteria don't need to be a source of bias if we interpret the findings appropriately. Bias can arise if we overinterpret or fail to understand the limitations of the data source. In fact, no data source is without potential sources of bias. A data user should always be able to explain who is *not* included, and how this could affect results.

For example, it is common to loosely interpret YRBSS findings as applying to all teenagers. In fact, YRBSS surveys teenagers who are attending a participating high school; it was designed to monitor the impact of school-based health programs. Not all schools or districts participate in YRBSS. To correctly interpret YRBSS data and its applicability to a local population, you should know which schools participate and how nonparticipating schools differ from participating schools. Individual students are also excluded for various reasons, including absence due to illness, dropping out, and language barriers. Parental permission policies vary, from being allowed to opt out if they don't want their children to participate to being required to opt in to allow their children to participate, obviously affecting the response rate and probably the representativeness of the sample. For these reasons, YRBSS may not be appropriate for assessing policies to help at-risk teens or for understanding the drivers of under-enrollment.

Hospital discharge data are another example of an existing data source that can be valuable for public health decision making but needs to be used carefully. Collected by hospitals for billing purposes, the data are compiled by state hospital associations and shared with researchers in various ways.[44] Hospital discharge data systems can describe inpatient stays, outpatient stays, and emergency department visits. They record patient demographics, diagnoses, procedures performed, and charges. Importantly, they exclude people who have not had encounters with hospital systems. Since most births occur in hospitals, hospitals can be a valid data source for studies of births. When hospital encounters are used to assess community health for issues like drug overdoses, asthma, or heart disease, bias can arise because of who is included and why. For example, we need to consider whether a population of interest might have fewer hospital admissions because they don't have the illness, because they are ill but receive outpatient care that keeps them from needing hospitalization, or because they have limited or no access to care.

The way a survey is administered can bias a study if the mode of delivery (e.g., mail, in person, phone, online) is less accessible or acceptable to some subpopulations. Disparities in response rates are common. For example, rural Native Americans may prefer face-to-face interviews to telephone surveys.[45] In one large study, older adults were more likely to respond to web- and mail-based surveys than to telephone surveys, and Black and Hispanic people had higher response rates when web and phone response options were included.[46] If a surveillance system depends on voluntary response, nonresponse bias is a common problem. This is true of some disease registries, government public health surveys, and most primary data collection surveys. Nonresponse bias occurs when response rates vary according to factors that are related to what we're trying to measure, such as socioeconomic or health status. Differential nonresponse or differential reporting can cause bias that is difficult to detect.

PRIVACY AND SOVEREIGNTY

Not all limitations of secondary data are because of characteristics of the data. A major barrier to utilization of some sources is limited access.[47] To protect patient privacy, datasets are de-identified[48] and there are serious legal consequences for institutions that disclose datasets containing identifiers. Identifiers include specifics such as name and date of birth, but they also include information that may seem less personal, such as the county of residence. Government public health entities need identifiers to perform functions such as surveillance and program planning, and there are exemptions from privacy laws for use of data by those entities.[49,50] States and other data owners have different interpretations of these laws, however, and in practice, local, tribal, and even state public health agencies sometimes cannot gain access at all or can't gain access in a timely manner. Data owners may fear that public health agencies do not have the capacity, time, or expertise to use and protect the data appropriately. Further, much public health work is done by nongovernmental agencies, which may need special legal agreements to use these data. Clearly defining data governance structures in advance can alleviate this problem.[51]

The authors have observed that when communities possess access to their own data, they can feel more empowered to plan and implement changes. If they can fully interrogate the data, they have more confidence in what it does (and does not) tell them, and more confidence in their own decisions. If they have ongoing access rather than receiving annual summary data from the data owners or a third party, they are more empowered to use it to monitor quality improvement projects and evaluate programs. It can be argued from an ethical point of view that the data *about* a community should be owned *by* the community. This concept of data sovereignty does not mean that every individual in the community sees data about other individuals, but instead that their representative public health agency, the part of their government that most directly serves the community, would have access. Public health agencies may also need to build technical capacity and allocate sufficient time to use the data in collaboration with and for the benefit of the community.

The rules and regulations regarding data sharing vary significantly by location, data source, and data user. Some states make data available more readily than others, and some have developed data access hubs that de-identify and securely link datasets together, making data not only more available but also more useful.[52] Whether you are collecting your own data or gathering existing data, it is important you understand data privacy requirements, including what protections are required to store it and how it can and can't be used. Seeking out these answers is something that should be prioritized at the data selection stage of any project. Institutional Review Boards are an important resource for public health practice as well as research, and Institutional Review Board approval is needed for publishing in most peer-reviewed journals.

REFERENCES

1. Clinical and Translational Science Awards Consortium Community Engagement Key Function Committee Task Force on the Principles of Community Engagement. *Principles of Community Engagement.* 2nd ed. June 2011. Accessed March 4, 2024. https://ictr.johnshopkins.edu/wp-content/uploads/2015/10/CTSAPrinciplesofCommunityEngagement.pdf
2. GenerateHealth. Accessed March 4, 2024. https://generatehealthstl.org
3. Brown HL, Smith M, Beasley Y, Conard T, Musselman AL, Caine VA. Infant mortality lessons learned from a fetal and infant mortality review program. *Matern Child Health J.* 2017;21(suppl 1):107–113. doi:10.1007/s10995-017-2384-y
4. National Center for Fatality Review & Prevention. *Fetal and Infant Mortality Review Manual: A Guide for Communities.* 2021. Accessed March 4, 2024. https://ncfrp.org/wp-content/uploads/NCRPCD-Docs/FIMRManual.pdf
5. Cochrane Library. Cochrane reviews. Accessed March 4, 2024. https://www.cochranelibrary.com
6. Littell JH, White H. The Campbell Collaboration: Providing better evidence for a better world. *Res Soc Work Pract.* 2018;28(1):6–12. doi:10.1177/1049731517703748
7. US Dept of Health and Human Services. Agency for Healthcare Research and Quality. Accessed March 4, 2024. https://www.ahrq.gov
8. The University of York. Centre for Reviews and Dissemination. Accessed March 4, 2024. https://www.york.ac.uk/crd
9. Community Preventive Services Task Force. The Guide to Community Preventive Services (The Community Guide). 2016. Accessed March 4, 2024. https://www.thecommunityguide.org
10. Odedina, FT, Stern, MC. Role of funders in addressing the continued lack of diversity in science and medicine. *Nat Med.* 2021;27:1859–1861. doi:10.1038/s41591-021-01555-8
11. Centre for Evidence-Based Medicine. Catalogue of bias. Accessed March 4, 2024. https://catalogofbias.org/biases
12. Ayorinde AA, Williams I, Mannion R, et al. Publication and related biases in health services research: A systematic review of empirical evidence. *BMC Med Res Methodol.* 2020;20:137. doi:10.1186/s12874-020-01010-1
13. Centers for Disease Control and Prevention. CDC data. Accessed October 29, 2024. https://data.cdc.gov/browse
14. US General Services Administration. Data.gov. Accessed October 28, 2024. https://data.gov
15. Mercer A, Lau A, Kennedy C. 1. How different weighting methods work. Pew Research Center. January 26, 2018. Accessed February 8, 2024. https://www.pewresearch.org/methods/2018/01/26/how-different-weighting-methods-work
16. Zhang X, Holt JB, Lu H, et al. Multilevel regression and poststratification for small-area estimation of population health outcomes: A case study of chronic obstructive pulmonary disease prevalence using the Behavioral Risk Factor Surveillance System. *Am J Epidemiol.* 2014;179(8):1025–1033. doi:10.1093/aje/kwu018
17. National Institutes of Health. List of registries. Updated January 6, 2025. Accessed March 4, 2024. https://www.nih.gov/health-information/nih-clinical-research-trials-you/list-registries

18. Blumenthal S. The use of clinical registries in the United States: A landscape survey. *EGEMS (Wash DC)*. 2017;5(1):26. doi:10.5334/egems.248
19. Centers for Disease Control and Prevention. National Notifiable Diseases Surveillance System. Updated November 20, 2024. Accessed February 6, 2025. https://www.cdc.gov/nndss/index.html
20. Centers for Disease Control and Prevention. CDC WONDER. Updated February 5, 2025. Accessed February 6, 2025. https://wonder.cdc.gov
21. McCarthy D. State all-payer claims databases: Tools for improving health care value, part 1. The Commonwealth Fund. December 10, 2020. Accessed March 4, 2024. https://www.commonwealthfund.org/publications/fund-reports/2020/dec/state-apcds-part-1-establish-make-functional
22. Children's Hospital Association. Leverage your data with CHA's Pediatric Health Information System. Accessed March 5, 2024. https://www.childrenshospitals.org/content/analytics/product-program/pediatric-health-information-system
23. Garza M, Del Fiol G, Tenenbaum J, Walden A, Nahm Zozus M. Evaluating common data models for use with a longitudinal community registry. *J Biomed Inform*. 2016;64:333–341. doi:10.1016/j.jbi.2016.10.016
24. Dixon BE, Grannis SJ, McAndrews C, et al. Leveraging data visualization and a statewide health information exchange to support COVID-19 surveillance and response: Application of public health informatics. *J Am Med Inform Assoc*. 2021;28(7)1363–1373. doi:10.1093/jamia/ocab004
25. Centers for Disease Control and Prevention. Youth online: high school YRBS. 2017. Accessed March 4, 2024. https://nccd.cdc.gov/youthonline/App/Default.aspx
26. Centers for Disease Control and Prevention. PLACES: Local data for better health. March 8, 2021. Accessed March 4, 2024. https://www.cdc.gov/PLACES
27. US Census Bureau. Small Area Income and Poverty Estimates (SAIPE) Program. October 5, 2018. Updated July 1, 2022. Accessed March 4, 2024. https://www.census.gov/programs-surveys/saipe.html
28. IPUMS. 2019. Accessed March 4, 2024. https://www.ipums.org
29. Boston University School of Social Work. Diversitydatakids.org. Accessed March 4, 2024. https://www.diversitydatakids.org
30. Health Resources and Services Administration. Data downloads. Accessed March 5, 2024. https://data.hrsa.gov/data/download?hmpgtitle=hmpg-hrsa-data
31. The Annie E. Casey Foundation. KIDS COUNT Data Center. Accessed March 4, 2024. https://datacenter.aecf.org
32. County Health Rankings & Roadmaps. Methodology and sources. Accessed March 5, 2024. https://www.countyhealthrankings.org/health-data/methodology-and-sources
33. Centers for Disease Control and Prevention. Community planning for health assessment: Data & benchmarks. Updated May 15, 2024. Accessed March 4, 2024. https://www.cdc.gov/public-health-gateway/php/public-health-strategy/public-health-strategies-for-community-health-assessment-data-benchmarks.html
34. National Institutes of Health. Repositories for sharing scientific data. Accessed March 4, 2024. https://sharing.nih.gov/data-management-and-sharing-policy/sharing-scientific-data/repositories-for-sharing-scientific-data

35. Kleinman, JC. Underreporting of infant deaths: Then and now. *Am J Public Health.* 1986;76(4):365–366. doi:10.2105/ajph.76.4.365
36. Jensen, E. Census Bureau expands focus on improving data for young children. February 10, 2022. Accessed March 4, 2024. https://www.census.gov/library/stories/2022/03/despite-efforts-census-undercount-of-young-children-persists.html
37. Wolff B, Mahoney F, Lohiniva AL, Corkum M. Collecting and analyzing qualitative data. In: Rasmussen SA, Goodman RA, eds. *The CDC Field Epidemiology Manual.* Centers for Disease Control and Prevention; 2018. Accessed March 4, 2024. https://www.cdc.gov/field-epi-manual/php/chapters/qualitative-data.html
38. National Center for Fatality Review & Prevention. Consulting population-based data to inform fetal and infant mortality review and community action decisions. June 2022. Accessed March 5, 2024. https://ncfrp.org/wp-content/uploads/Report_Population-Health-and-FIMR-Guidance.pdf
39. Kirchherr J, Charles K. Enhancing the sample diversity of snowball samples: Recommendations from a research project on anti-dam movements in Southeast Asia. *PLoS One.* 2018;13(8): e0201710. doi:10.1371/journal.pone.0201710
40. Handcock MS, Gile KJ. Comment: On the concept of snowball sampling. *Sociol Methodol.* 2011;41(1):367–371. doi:10.1111/j.1467-9531.2011.01243
41. Maddow-Zimet I, Kost K. Effect of changes in response options on reported pregnancy intentions: A natural experiment in the United States. *Public Health Rep.* 2020;135(3):354–363. doi:10.1177/0033354920914344
42. US Census Bureau. *American Community Survey and Puerto Rico Community Survey Design and Methodology Report.* November 2022. Accessed February 6, 2025. https://www.census.gov/programs-surveys/acs/methodology/design-and-methodology.html
43. Centers for Disease Control and Prevention. Youth Risk Behavior Surveillance System (YRBSS). Accessed February 14, 2025. https://www.cdc.gov/yrbs/index.html
44. Agency for Healthcare Research and Quality. Healthcare Cost and Utilization Project (HCUP). Updated January 2025. Accessed February 6, 2025. https://www.ahrq.gov/data/hcup/index.html
45. English KC, Espinoza J, Pete D, Tjemsland A. A comparative analysis of telephone and in-person survey administration for public health surveillance in rural American Indian communities. *J Public Health Manag Pract.* 2019;25(suppl 5):S70–S76. doi:10.1097/PHH.0000000000001007
46. Elliott MN, Brown JA, Hambarsoomian K, et al. Survey protocols, response rates, and representation of underserved patients: A randomized clinical trial. *JAMA Health Forum.* 2024;5(1): e234929. doi:10.1001/jamahealthforum.2023.4929
47. Macek C, Boillot N. Opinion: The hidden costs of data protection in public health. *Devex.* January 9, 2019. Accessed March 5, 2024. https://www.devex.com/news/opinion-the-hidden-costs-of-data-protection-in-public-health-94084
48. US Dept of Health and Human Services. Guidance regarding methods for de-identification of protected health information in accordance with the Health Insurance Portability and Accountability Act (HIPAA) Privacy Rule. September 7, 2012. Accessed March 4, 2024. https://www.hhs.gov/hipaa/for-professionals/privacy/special-topics/de-identification/index.html
49. US Dept of Health and Human Services. Disclosures for public health activities. Updated April 3, 2003. Accessed March 4, 2024. https://www.hhs.gov/hipaa/for-professionals/privacy/guidance/disclosures-public-health-activities/index.html

50. Lucido S, Koo D, Hodge JG Jr. HIPAA Privacy Rule and public health guidance from CDC and the US Department of Health and Human Services. *MMWR Morb Mortal Wkly Rep*. 2003;52: 1–12. Accessed March 4, 2024. https://www.cdc.gov/mmwr/preview/mmwrhtml/m2e411a1.htm
51. Griffiths KE, Blain J, Vajdic CM, Jorm L. Indigenous and tribal peoples' data governance in health research: A systematic review. *Int J Environ Res Public Health*. 2021;18(19):10318. doi:10.3390/ijerph181910318
52. Massachusetts Data Office. Massachusetts data hub. Accessed March 5, 2024. https://data.mass.gov

3

Data Analysis for Decision Making

The Centers for Disease Control and Prevention (CDC)'s online Introduction to Epidemiology[1] describes the purposes of public health as a matter of identifying causes of disease, risk factors for those diseases, and subpopulations most affected. The agency depicts its public health approach as a linear process that starts with those epidemiologic fact-finding steps and proceeds to evaluate and implement interventions that can address the problem (Figure 3-1).[1] The underlying assumption seems to be that we trust our surveillance systems to keep us informed, and we use analysis to allocate resources.

Reality is not as simple. Identification of common problems can be accomplished through routine surveillance of populations, as depicted in Figure 3-1. But we must also identify emerging issues that we don't expect, root causes, and, of course, solutions that are tailored to our community's needs. This means that routine surveillance must be accompanied by creative use of the data sources at our disposal. These include data from our own programs, systems that study sentinel events, and feedback from community members such as agency heads, frontline workers, and consumers of health services. Identifying an appropriate intervention is not as easy as one would hope. Though programs abound, rigorous evaluations do not, and even evaluated programs can't be successfully replicated everywhere. In real communities, powerful contextual factors such as environment, socioeconomics, leadership, and culture must be considered in any meaningful problem analysis or evaluation. The public health field has learned that *community involvement* is a key ingredient for success in identifying, describing, and solving problems.

This chapter does not cover statistical methods or epidemiology— that would require several college courses. Instead, it is an overview of the kind of thinking that public health practitioners need when they want to use data and information to guide action. The authors recommend that health departments use surveillance systems routinely and continuously to alert public health leaders to urgent needs, disparities, or alarming trends. However, some conditions are not detected by these systems, and data alone do not necessarily lead to action. Public health departments that maintain close, ongoing relationships with people in the communities they serve will be more successful at identifying problems and engaging the community in solving them.

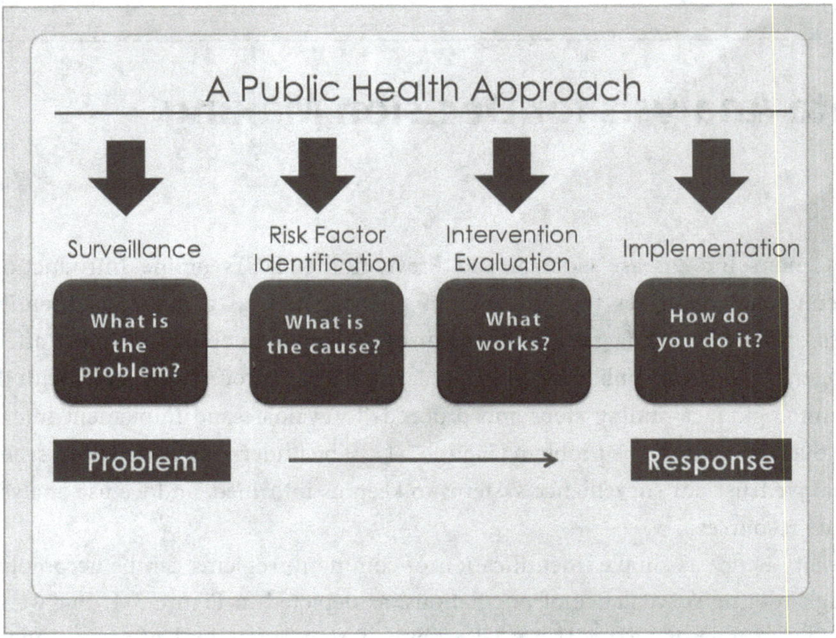

Source: Reprinted from Centers for Disease Control and Prevention.[1]

Figure 3-1. A Public Health Approach

GUIDING PRINCIPLES

We begin with a set of guiding principles that can help steer communities and health departments through the complex task of identifying, understanding, and addressing health problems in their jurisdictions. We assume that analysts work with a "community group" to keep the analytic and planning processes grounded in the practical realities of relevant populations and systems. The goal of this chapter is to help you analyze problems with the help of all available information, including data of all types and knowledge of the community, so you can "make the case" to funders and guide policymakers to implement the right changes. Box 3-1 introduces the five principles that should be used to guide these analyses.

1. Clearly Understand the Purpose of the Analysis

Be clear on the purpose of gathering and/or using the data. Identify the agenda(s) and positionality of your agency, funders, and other partners, including those who will do the analyses (see principle 4 in Box 3-1), by thinking through the following types of questions. If we are trying to identify priorities, whose priorities will they be, who will be at the table, and what will be the criteria? If we need the data for a grant application or

Box 3-1. Five Guiding Principles of Analysis

1. Clearly understand the purpose of the analysis.
2. Examine the relevant causal relationships and question all assumptions.
3. Consult complementary information sources while recognizing the value of many kinds of information.
4. Assume your information has bias and identify its sources (human, systems, and data).
5. Follow the "nothing about us without us" rule by including your subjects on your analytic team.

report, what is the goal of the grant? What is the funder's goal? What are the goals of the population that the funded program serves? If we are doing research, are we clear about the question we are trying to answer (see principles 2 and 3)? If this is part of ongoing surveillance, is there a trigger mechanism for action? Are we following principle 5? If this is a special study, is there a funder or policymaker with an agenda to advocate for a particular change? What populations are we trying to address and why? Is there a benchmark goal or comparison population for our outcome(s)?

2. Examine the Relevant Causal Relationships and Question All Assumptions

There are many possible causes, contributors, and confounders that could be affecting a particular population's health outcome. We must consider all these factors, rather than focusing on just one or two because they are included in our main data source or because they have been used traditionally. We need to include relationships supported by the scientific literature, such as "smoking causes cancer" or "receiving formula samples in the hospital discourages breastfeeding." Making cause-and-effect diagrams, known as directed acyclic graphs,[2] during group brainstorming sessions can help everyone visualize the complex systems that may be involved and elicit ideas from various perspectives. Consider both positive and negative influences, factors that act on individual, community, and policy levels, and the perspectives of multiple sectors. These simple diagrams created by groups can be used for building valid analytic models and can contribute to logic models as programs are developed.

3. Consult Complementary Information Sources While Recognizing the Value of Many Kinds of Information

Using complementary information sources rather than relying on one source or one kind of analysis is critical. This means not only including population-based quantitative data but also understanding the scientific literature, which sometimes identifies causal relationships among the things we measure. This means incorporating findings from local surveys, qualitative studies, and case review processes. These add detail, context, and causes that are not measured in surveillance systems. It also means seeking out expert opinions from other organizations within your jurisdiction, from federal agencies, and especially from community members who contribute their personal experience and knowledge of the community.

4. Assume Your Information Has Bias and Identify Its Sources (Human, Systems, and Data)

Analytic methods rest on assumptions that are seldom fully met, and each study has many decision points that are subject to the biases of the decision makers. Rather than pretending we and our data are objective, it is good practice to seek out and identify potential sources of bias and then work to mitigate their effects. Analytically, we can use distribution-free or nonparametric methods and sensitivity analyses, we can repeat or redesign the analysis with a different data source or over-sample from underrepresented groups, and we can use appropriate imputation methods for missing data. Because our analytic decisions are influenced by our own biases, we can also examine our backgrounds and positionality, include people with different perspectives as decision makers, use tools and exercises that have been developed to identify bias (see the Good Science Demands We Identify Sources of Bias in Data and Take Steps to Minimize Their Impact section later), and be transparent about our assumptions.

5. Follow the "Nothing About Us Without Us" Rule by Including Your Subjects on Your Analytic Team

We can use the "nothing about us without us" principle. This means including people from the communities we are trying to assist, as well as the multisector professionals who serve them. For example, if you are investigating low health care access in a neighborhood, find ways to learn about the experiences and opinions of people from that neighborhood and the providers who seek to serve them. If you are evaluating a health department program, include program participants and program staff in planning the evaluation and interpreting the findings. We can include community members as advisors or researchers in analysis planning and interpretation and in decision making. Recognize that positionality and power differences can discourage or limit needed participation.

GOOD SCIENCE

The five principles previously discussed are fundamental and will lead to better decisions, but we recognize the extra work that following these principles will take. Improving scientific rigor usually slows down any process, and public health agencies are chronically under-resourced and often understaffed. However, a more inclusive analysis and planning process can lead to more sound conclusions, better acceptance of decisions, faster and more effective implementation of needed changes, and, ultimately, improved health outcomes. It is critical to remember that accurate data analysis relies upon practicing *good science*. The remainder of this chapter walks us through several considerations that help to ensure this high standard.

Good Science Requires Preparation

If you are working in or contracting for a government health department, you should prepare by connecting or reconnecting with existing community groups. Most communities have coalitions or collaboratives working on general or specific issues. Meeting with these groups or convening multiple groups to consider your problem area would show respect for the work already ongoing and help get you and your agency up to speed. If existing groups don't already include lay members of the community, take on the responsibility of making this happen. Use your time with community groups to both give and receive information. Because of your governmental positioning, you are likely to have access to secondary data that they lack. Because secondary data sources are, by nature, limited in scope, having collaborators with lived experience can keep you grounded and aware of important issues that existing data sources don't measure. The "nothing about us without us" principle demands that we keep pushing for more relevant information rather than having our thinking limited by the data at hand.

As a practical reality, government health departments need full and ongoing access to data about their populations so they can monitor health, investigate problems, and recommend appropriate interventions. However, many state, local, and tribal health agencies do not have ready access to key secondary data sources, even though federal law permits the use of data protected by the Health Insurance Portability and Accountability Act (HIPAA) for public health purposes.[3] Early in the process, learn about administrative and legal barriers and start addressing them to ensure you have access to the facts you need to be responsive to community decision makers. Build and strengthen systems that allow ongoing, routine access to a variety of sources for monitoring your population's health, access to health care, and social factors that impact these measures. One way to gain access is to collaborate with agencies who do have access, such as a "data division" within your agency, insurance companies, or health care systems. If your agency or collaborators do not have the capacity to analyze secondary data files, ensure that your relationship with the data owner allows timely access to tailored summary information with full transparency regarding data quality issues.

Good Science Means Knowing Your Data Before You Begin Your Analysis

Learn about the data sources and their limitations (see Chapter 2). Obtain specific details on how the respondents were selected, response rates, weighting, the meaning of each variable, who collected the information and entered the data, and how it was collected (direct measurement such as a lab result, self-report, informant, face-to-face versus online, or other details). Learn the rules and the exceptions. For example, birth certificate forms have a section that is filled out by the baby's parent, but what happens if the parent is ill or doesn't speak English? Are parents made aware that they can check more than one box to indicate their race, and yet another box for ethnicity? For data items taken from the medical record, such as prenatal care, how does care received in a different hospital affect the data and your analysis? Finding flaws in the data collection system doesn't mean you can't use the data, but it gives you the opportunity to adjust and be transparent. Finding flaws may also motivate efforts to improve the data collection processes. Another way to know your data is to begin by exploring *fully disaggregated* data and being intentional about how you aggregate and categorize. Initial checks for logical inconsistency and univariate and bivariate descriptive analysis, including plots of individual points, can save you from serious analytic mistakes. Common mistakes include failing to detect patterns such as truncation or outliers that could indicate data entry or coding problems or inadvertently erasing disparities by combining high-risk and low-risk groups. Another mistake is to create models based on unsupported combinations. For example, if your jurisdiction-based dataset includes very few immigrants with high educational attainment, then your dataset will not support a study about whether immigrants with master's degrees are more likely to access cancer screening services. Response rates for key study variables that aren't part of the dataset's weighting scheme should be assessed because nonresponse to a survey item can be correlated with its true value. For example, people who experience domestic violence may be less likely to answer a question designed to assess its prevalence than people who have not, which would bias your estimate downward. If data are collected at different locations or facilities, bivariate analyses may reveal differences in reporting processes. Statistical tests can estimate the likelihood of obtaining the variation shown by your data if reporting processes are indeed consistent, helping you to detect inconsistency. The people who perform the data collection or data cleaning may be able to explain differences based on their processes and limitations.

Good Science Demands We Identify Sources of Bias in Data and Take Steps to Minimize Their Impact

Hopefully, reading Chapter 2 has made you suspect bias in every data source and has given you some tools for identifying it. Data can be biased whether it is collected for your project (primary) or you are using an existing source (secondary). Investigators are also biased, and our biases influence the way we use data. Every analytic process has many assumptions and decision points, from what questions we ask and who we study, to what data we select or collect, to which methods we use for analysis. Each decision is subject to the biases of the decision makers. Positionality statements (see Chapter 1) help you and your readers identify your biases. Using positionality statements and other tools can also help you recognize the choices you are making in any study, and even potentially change your choices.

The concept of recognizing decisions and their biases is promoted and taught by We All Count, a "project for equity and data science" and a resource we recommend.[4] The We All Count authors developed a tool they call the Perspective Microscope (Figure 3-2), for examining a problem from multiple perspectives.[4,5] Exploring multiple perspectives can encourage investigators to integrate multiple research questions and data sources into an assessment rather than limiting ourselves to what we have done before or what is in our dataset. In the microscope exercise, the **eyepiece** at the top of the microscope represents the perspective from which the problem is observed; the **lens** represents the issue or goal at hand; and the **sample** being examined represents the data source. Consider a project to assess childhood asthma in your city. The analyst first lists the entities or systems that play a role, such as the mayor, hospitals, insurance companies, residents, and the housing authority. If the mayor is at the eyepiece and hospitals are the source of data, we might ask how many children visited emergency rooms for asthma in the past year. If the hospitals are at the eyepiece and pharmaceutical records

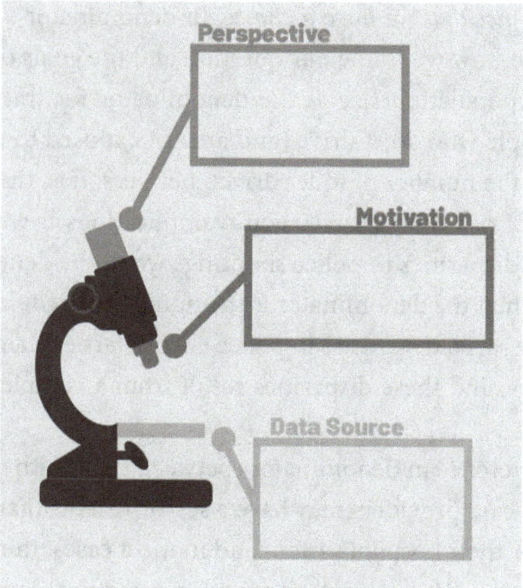

Source: Reprinted from We All Count.[4]

Figure 3-2. The Perspective Microscope Exercise

are the data source, we might ask whether parents and children are using medication appropriately. If the children's perspective is centered and the housing authority is the data source, we could ask about the availability of safe, affordable housing. Which perspective is the most important? It may be that we need all three (or more) to fully understand the issues and opportunities for improvement. We certainly don't want to assume there is only one perspective based on our funding source or which data source is most accessible to us. Even if we don't have the resources to study all perspectives immediately, being aware of others can open possibilities and put them on our agenda for future study to seek better solutions.

Good Science Means Using the Right Denominator

Our perspective can also be reflected in our choice of denominator. A simple rule in epidemiology is that the denominator is the population at risk of having the outcome we are concerned about. In most studies, we must consider the population at risk to make sense of a problem. It would be meaningless to compare the number of infant deaths in Omaha with the number in Los Angeles because of the enormous difference in the numbers of births, so we divide the number of deaths by the correct denominator, the number of births, to create comparable rates. The correct denominator can be the whole population, such as the total number of births, or it can be the count of a subpopulation. For example, we would measure short birth spacing only for the population of pregnant people who had a previous birth, because first-time births aren't at risk for this outcome.

The choice, *or the fact that we have a choice,* in denominator selection is not always clear. It can depend on how we frame our question and the goals of our investigation or messaging. If we use population size as the denominator for traffic fatalities, then for places with many people who don't drive (and are not exposed to the risk), rates will be artificially low. Using the number of miles driven per person as the denominator gives a more direct measure of risk. There can be equity implications as well. For example, studies tend to find racial disparities in police shootings when the denominator is the whole population, but not when the denominator is the number of people who had encounters with the police.[6] Large racial disparities in police encounters explain the difference in the incidence of shootings, and these disparities result from a complex web of current and historical causes.[7]

There is often a difference in denominators between the health care and public health points of view: health care providers may have a set of patients that is attributed to them by insurance payers or their hospital system and in most cases, this is not the same population as the residents of the health department jurisdiction. The health care denominator works well for measuring the quality of care among people who see the provider, but when we consider social determinants of health, public health wants to consider everyone in the jurisdiction, whether they have a family doctor or not.[8] In fact, populations without a strong connection to the health care system are usually a high priority for public health. When population size (or density) is causally related to the outcome, as in some infectious disease scenarios, it may need to be modeled as a confounder rather than a denominator.[9]

Good Science Involves Diagramming the Problem

Before setting up a model for your analysis, use diagramming to map out how you believe the different forces influence the outcome. Go through this process with your analytic team, and again with different community groups. Such diagrams are often called directed acyclic graphs, or DAGs.[2,10] They include factors that are thought to be causes, but also factors that interact with causes, modifying their effect, and factors that are confounders because they contribute to both cause and effect. An example DAG is shown in Figure 3-3 depicting the role of low birth weight in the association between perinatal risk factors and infant mortality.[11,12] Diagramming helps identify assumptions and can prevent serious analytic errors. There is often the temptation to "control for" everything in our dataset that could affect the outcome, without really thinking through how each data element is related to the outcome and exposure of interest. In an example one of the authors encountered, a project designed to determine if living in a food desert impacted a child's likelihood of experiencing hospitalization, socioeconomic status (SES) was added as a related factor to control for. Adjusting for this variable *completely eliminated* the association between living in a food desert and pediatric hospitalizations, leading to the conclusion that living in a food desert had no impact on pediatric hospitalization when accounting for the SES of the child. This analysis missed the point of investigating the relationship of interest. If the team had fully diagrammed the problem first, they would have considered SES an effect modifier rather than a confounder, as one's SES would affect one's ability to seek food sources outside of one's immediate area. A model stratified by SES would have allowed them to investigate the relationship of interest. DAGs can incorporate published scientific evidence about cause-and-effect relationships as well as the experience-based beliefs of the people constructing them. Engaging community groups in the diagramming process can identify factors and causal connections that the analyst or agency had not considered.[13] If community groups identify important factors that are not represented in traditional data sources, other data sources can be sought, or new data can be gathered. This interactive process can help identify and build consensus around the analytic assumptions. DAGs can also help interpret the analytic findings and may help guide the selection of program and systems changes.

A key assumption that many statistical methods are based on, "independent and identically distributed units of analysis," is seldom met in human populations. People are

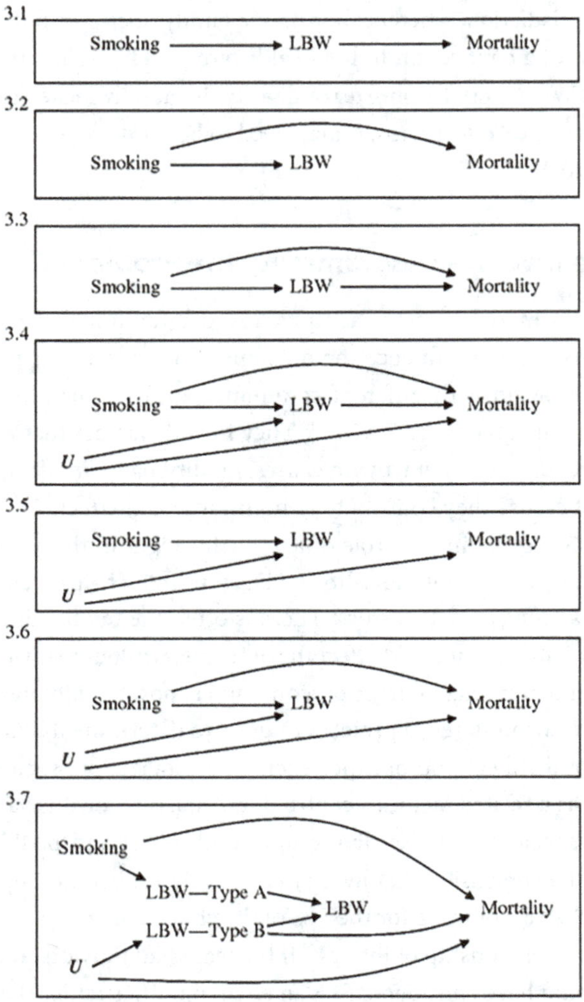

Source: Hernández-Díaz et al.[12] Reprinted with permission of Oxford University Press.
Note: LBW = low birth weight; U = other unmeasured risk factors (e.g., birth defects).

Figure 3-3. Causal Structure (Directed Acyclic Graph) Proposed to Represent the Role of Low Birth Weight in the Association Between Perinatal Risk Factors and Infant Mortality

often biologically related to others in their community, and their beliefs and behaviors are influenced by their common environments and social interactions in person and via media. Distributional assumptions such as normality also may not be met in practice. Fortunately, scientists are aware of this situation, and methods exist for analyzing correlated data and testing hypotheses using robust statistics (which are likely to produce correct results under a variety of assumptions). Epidemiologists can learn and employ these methods. For example, continuous data that is not normally distributed, like most time variables (such as length of hospital stay) can be analyzed using nonparametric tests. When observations are correlated within groups (e.g., children of the same parent, patients with the same primary care provider, multiple hospitalizations by the same person), the analyst can either account for this correlation by using mixed effects models or they can limit the analysis to one observation per group (e.g., only include one child per parent, only include the first hospitalization per patient). If it is not clear which way a particular variable or situation should be modeled, a sensitivity analysis can be run with an alternative model.

Good Science Partners With Community Members

Fostering good relationships between the community and their data can improve data use. People who collect and analyze data can meet over time with community groups, learning about their concerns and perspectives, introducing them to the available data sources and measures, and learning and addressing concerns they might have about validity and meaning. Unsubstantiated concerns can be addressed by increasing understanding. Valid concerns usually indicate that the data need to be interpreted with caution rather than being thrown out entirely. If community members feel that a question on a survey is likely to be misunderstood, the analyst may be able to pose alternate findings based on *either* interpretation so the community can see the potential impact of the poorly worded question. Consider one of many examples of discovering, validating, and moving forward despite underlying data quality concerns. Community meetings with hospital system representatives might reveal systematic data collection differences; if one hospital has a policy of following up with each very low-birth-weight delivery to determine whether the baby was discharged alive or received a death certificate, and a second hospital does not follow up,[11] the first hospital would appear to have a higher death rate among babies born with a very low birth weight. This would make comparisons of very low-birth-weight mortality rates biased and invalid but might not significantly affect overall comparisons of infant mortality. Transparency about the limitations of the data can boost community confidence. A mutual understanding of data findings as signposts or guardrails rather than complete information can ensure that the community's knowledge is incorporated into the decision making process.

The process of diagramming a problem and its contributors, as described in the previous section, provides an excellent vehicle to help researchers learn from the perspectives of a variety of community members. Helping formulate diagrams of problems and causes allows people with no statistical training to contribute to the analytic modeling process. Further, community members can assist with the design of surveys or discussion questions for collection of primary data. They could also participate as survey respondents or key informants.

Community members can be engaged for input on how disparities should be calculated and displayed to the public. It isn't always constructive to simply show prevalence for each group, especially when the pattern is similar for many outcomes. The focus community can feel targeted rather than prioritized, and there is evidence that the public does indeed tend to blame the victim for disparities.[14] Alternatives include comparing each group to an agreed-upon goal or reference population. An advantage of using a reference population rather than a simple numeric goal is that the reference population can be a real group of people that has already reached a goal. This group can be chosen so that it is meaningful from a political or funding perspective, to provide leverage to motivate change. It can also be powerful for public display to invert the problem and display only the gap, attributing it to failure of the relevant systems instead of to the population groups the systems have failed.[15] For example, instead of showing the prevalence of the health outcome of five racial groups in a bar chart and highlighting the difference between Whites and each other group, which is typical, display only the highest and lowest bar, labeling only the gap and naming some systems that contribute to it.

Good Science Centers the Priority Population

Traditionally, epidemiologists tend to divide their jurisdiction into pieces like a pie, comparing prevalence and risk factors across subgroups that must add up to the whole. Instead, we can focus on the priority population(s) one at a time. This allows us to include all the people in that group, even if they overlap (intersect) with other groups. This is often an issue for race and ethnicity, where most surveillance systems now allow people to check more than one choice. Reports often provide data for the single-race groups, combining multiracial people into one category. While the multiracial group may be a small population relative to the majority, it can be large compared with other small groups. This practice reduces the numbers in the smaller racial/ethnic groups and changes their composition. We recommend starting with communities and involving them in decisions on how groups should be aggregated.

One way that small groups get de-prioritized is by comparing the *P* values of multiple groups and prioritizing groups that are statistically significant. Because statistical significance depends on both the effect size (distance from the reference point) and the statistical power to detect a difference (which depends on sample size), groups that have the same effect size can have different *P* values. This often leads to potentially harmful conclusions like "the effect of the intervention was statistically significant for Blacks and Hispanics/Latines but insignificant for Native Americans." Rather than depending on statistical significance or *P* values for decision making, the authors recommend depicting actual effect sizes with confidence intervals or addressing the small numbers and statistical power as described below.

Small numbers in a population or sample can be problematic for several reasons. First, rates or proportions based on small numbers can vary widely from one time period to the next. This is true whether our data source includes the whole population or a sample, and we generally don't want to make big changes based on a rate that could double or halve the next time we check. The second problem occurs when numbers are so small that individuals can be identified. Privacy is extremely important. There are some good analytic alternatives that avoid ignoring or suppressing numbers for populations with small numbers. First, we may be able to expand the time frame or geographical area to obtain more reliable, if less specific, evidence. Second, we may be able to use a more specific and powerful statistical model or test, such as Fisher's exact test, for a particular population. Although epidemiologists may be accustomed to using complex statistical models to investigate causal relationships, causal inference isn't always what is needed when investigating a problem in a community. If causality has already been established in the literature and the goal is to identify vulnerable subgroups or predominant risk factors in the community, simpler analyses are often both statistically more powerful and more meaningful. Third, we can employ control charting methods that signal when system changes may be occurring and a response is warranted. Fourth, if our data source is a survey, we may be able to oversample from the underrepresented group to increase numbers. Finally, and perhaps always, we can use qualitative methods to understand the systems that impact health in the community. Case review methodologies that involve community members, such as fetal and infant mortality reviews, have for many years successfully identified needs and motivated systems changes based on very small numbers.

Good Science Links Datasets Together

It is likely that more than one data source will be needed to encompass all the factors that were identified as important in creation of the DAG. Luckily, data sources can typically be joined or linked together using common units of observation. If two or more of the datasets you wish to use have identifiers and you either have ethical access to those identifiers or access to hashing or tokenization software, then you can link the datasets at the individual level. It is common to have place-based data, such as neighborhood median income or an air quality measure, that can be added to an individual-level dataset. These can be "joined" on their geo-IDs. Geo-IDs are identifiers consisting of a sequence of numbers with smaller area-level codes joined to the identifiers of the larger area they belong to (i.e., county codes consist of the state's 2-digit code followed by a 3-digit code to specify the county within the state). If you want to link data from a smaller geographic unit to a larger one, you need to think carefully about how to aggregate. You will need to consider both the numerator and denominator of the data you are aggregating. For example, you might have a dataset with the rate of pediatric asthma hospitalizations per census tract and want to investigate the impact of traffic density, but you only have this information at the block group level. You will need to aggregate both the number of vehicles and the number of roads in the block groups to recalculate the average across the whole census tract that those block groups fit within.

Good Science Builds the Evidence Base

Public health practitioners can (and must) help build the evidence base by building evaluation into their interventions. In recent years, many funders have been including this as a requirement. Evaluations do add burden, but when designed with care, they can help you improve your programs *and* they can help other health departments learn what works. Perhaps the most important and most overlooked part of evaluations is describing both the context and the intervention in enough detail that it can be replicated and adapted to new contexts. Evaluations need a way to estimate what would have happened if the intervention hadn't been implemented. This can be done effectively using a control group, particularly if people in the control group are well matched with people in the intervention group. Self-selection, a common method for assigning people to groups in public health practice, often leads to differences between the control and intervention groups that are big enough to invalidate the study, but individual randomization is not always practical. Alternatives to control groups without individual randomization include statistically controlling for differences, group randomization, and using analytic methods like propensity score matching or network analysis. If having a separate control group is completely unfeasible, options include techniques like using data on initial condition from the same population (interrupted time series) and comparing outcomes in similar populations who either did not implement the intervention or implemented it at a different point in time (difference in difference). A key part of demonstrating that your intervention *caused* the change or difference is to identify the mechanisms for change (i.e., the actual causes of behavior or outcome changes). In communities, qualitative research can be a valuable tool for identifying mechanisms. Communities are where health issues are most acutely felt and where the energy for change is found. Solutions are implemented in communities and documenting these stories may be the best way to help other communities learn.

Good Science Synthesizes the Evidence

Even with the ability to link data and the many secondary data sources available, you will not be able to cover all important factors about a problem in a single analysis. However, you can knit together multiple analyses (both qualitative and quantitative) alongside what you found in the literature to derive a more complete picture. Going back to the diagram you made about the problem, map each analysis and piece of external literature back to each relationship that was determined to be important in your community. If you find that an important piece is still missing, comb back through your data resources and see if there are data that can be used to address it. If not, then this is a good potential factor in future primary data generation efforts. It is very important in this step, and in all steps, that your decisions about what data to pursue and further analyses to undertake incorporate the feedback of the different stakeholders involved. It is important to guard yourself against tendencies towards your own preferences and ideas of what is important.

REFERENCES

1. Centers for Disease Control and Prevention. Introduction to Public Health. 2014. Accessed March 4, 2024. https://www.cdc.gov/training-publichealth101/media/pdfs/introduction-to-public-health.pdf
2. Digitale JC, Martin JN, Glymour MM. Tutorial on directed acyclic graphs. *J Clin Epidemiol.* 2022;142:264–267. doi:10.1016/j.jclinepi.2021.08.001
3. Ramanathan T, Schmit C, Akshara M, Dawn P, Gregory S, Matthew P. Federal public health laws supporting data use and sharing. Centers for Disease Control and Prevention. March 19, 2015. Accessed March 4, 2024. https://stacks.cdc.gov/view/cdc/44666
4. We All Count. About us. Accessed March 4, 2024. https://weallcount.com/about-us
5. We All Count. Foundations of data equity tool guide. 2022. Accessed March 4, 2024. https://weallcount.com/wp-content/uploads/2022/02/Foundations-of-Data-Equity-Tool-Guide.pdf
6. Tregle B, Nix J, Alpert GP. Disparity does not mean bias: Making sense of observed racial disparities in fatal officer-involved shootings with multiple benchmarks. *J Crime Justice.* 2018;42(1):18–31. doi:10.1080/0735648X.2018.1547269
7. Muhammad KG. *The Condemnation of Blackness: Race, Crime, and the Making of Modern Urban America.* Harvard University Press; 2019.
8. Calman NS, Hauser D, Chokshi DA. "Lost to follow-up": The public health goals of accountable care. *Arch Intern Med.* 2012;172(7):584–586. doi:10.1001/archinternmed.2012.219
9. Morrison CN, Rundle AG, Branas CC, Chihuri S, Mehranbod C, Li G. The unknown denominator problem in population studies of disease frequency. *Spat Spatiotemporal Epidemiol.* 2020;35:100361. doi:10.1016/j.sste.2020.100361
10. Subiza-Peréz M, García-Baquero G, Fernández-Somoano A, et al. Social inequalities, green and blue spaces and mental health in 6–12 years old children participating in the INMA cohort. *Health Place.* 2023;83:103104. doi:10.1016/j.healthplace.2023.103104
11. Kleinman JC. Underreporting of infant deaths: Then and now. *Am J Public Health.* 1986;76(4):365–366. doi:10.2105/ajph.76.4.365
12. Hernández-Díaz S, Schisterman EF, Hernán MA. The birth weight "paradox" uncovered? *Am J Epidemiol.* 2006;164(11):1115–1120. doi:10.1093/aje/kwj275
13. Krause H, Richburg-Hayes L. The Data Equity Framework: A concrete and systematic equity-oriented approach to quantitative data projects. *SocArXiv.* Preprint posted online March 23, 2023. doi:10.31235/osf.io/sqt4u

14. Roundtable on Population Health Improvement; Board on Population Health and Public Health Practice; Health and Medicine Division; National Academies of Sciences, Engineering, and Medicine. *Framing the Dialogue on Race and Ethnicity to Advance Health Equity: Proceedings of a Workshop*. National Academies Press; 2016.
15. Castillo W, Gillborn D. How to "QuantCrit:" Practices and questions for education data researchers and users. *EdWorkingPapers (Brown University)*. Preprint posted online September 2023. doi:10.26300/v5kh-dd65

4

Building Consensus and Reaching Decisions

Throughout this book, we have discussed the use of data in public health action, arguing that data should inform our actions and be a catalyst for community conversations about health. We have also outlined multiple data sources and overviewed several analytic techniques aimed at revealing important patterns and key nuances in the data. In this chapter, we shift our attention to building consensus through data and ultimately reaching broadly supported decisions. To do this, we provide real-world examples of instances when public health actions resulted in significant social strains and strive to identify what went wrong. We also apply Daniel Goleman's emotional intelligence model[1] to develop a series of key considerations that public health professionals can follow to avoid unnecessary conflicts.

IS CONSENSUS POSSIBLE?

Reaching consensus on public health activities can be a significant challenge. Through our various roles in research and practice, the authors have witnessed and participated in countless public health planning efforts in dozens of cities across the United States. Without exception, all these efforts have encountered disagreement—most minor, but many significant and longstanding. Because of this, adept data usage requires more than technical intelligence with aspects of data collection and analysis. It also necessitates exceptional emotional intelligence, which is defined as the ability to "recognize and regulate emotions in ourselves and in others."[2(p14)] That definition makes clear that the work of emotional intelligence involves not only personal but also social aspects of recognizing and appropriately responding to emotional dynamics.

Too often, we overlook the importance of emotional intelligence in the practice of public health, but there is no denying the work is *social* in nature. We serve as public stewards, entrusted with our communities' most vital resource—health. In addition to this, many of us are employed by governmental entities. Mishandling of public relationships and social gaffes can lead to breakdowns in trust between community members and public health officials. At their worst, these breakdowns can lead to open animosity and stymie attempts to improve adverse health outcomes.

Case #1: Sleeping with Knives

Unfortunately, breakdowns in trust between public health officials and the communities they serve are nothing new.[3] For this reason, we should carefully consider instances where conflict has emerged and see what lessons can be learned to improve our ability to manage community relations through the process of data-informed decision making. Consider a case from a midwestern local health department, which wanted to reduce high infant mortality rates in their community. The data told them that co-sleeping deaths were a significant driver of their elevated rates, so they hired a marketing firm to design a public campaign. On bus stops and billboards around the city, they displayed images of babies sleeping with butcher knives along with the caption: "Your baby sleeping with you can be just as dangerous."

Prior to launch, the health department shared the campaign with other public health experts around the nation and received positive feedback and even requests for the digital files to replicate the campaign in their communities. However, when the images went up, many residents were appalled. They felt the campaign had crossed a line and was insulting to parents who chose to co-sleep and took efforts to do so safely, wanting to enhance parent–infant bonding, improve breastfeeding, reduce postpartum depression, and receive a host of other possible benefits. When confronted with public outcry, the health department stood firm, insisting the practice of co-sleeping was dangerous. They even cited a case of a local infant death due to co-sleeping just prior to the launch of the campaign and noted that 30 other nations had better infant mortality rates than their community. However, opponents pointed out that co-sleeping is the norm in many of these nations and infant sleep isolation (as it is sometimes known) is considered harmful.[4,5]

This case illustrates the point that as public health professionals, we can have the best intentions but not always realize optimal outcomes. Our aims may be based on data and aligned with established public health practices. They may even be lauded by other public health professionals and backed up by key standards such as Healthy People 2030 or respected agencies such as the World Health Organization. However, the "public" moniker in our name necessitates that our methods are supported by the communities we serve and are carried out in ways that are equitable and respectful.

As you reflect on this case, ask yourself which side, if any, you identify with most. The health department's campaign was undeniably successful in capturing the attention of the public and shining a light on the issue of co-sleeping. But was it effective at changing behavior? Moreover, was the health department's data-driven goal to prevent co-sleeping correct, or should it have been aiming to mitigate the risks of a practice that many community members found advantageous?

In considering these questions, it is important to remember that there are also many examples of "opinion-driven" decisions (i.e., health decisions not supported by data) that cause bad outcomes. For example, there were once pervasive and strong opinions that bottle feeding was better than breastfeeding. Data demonstrated that this was not the case and eventually public opinion shifted to align with the data. Additionally, segments of the public continue to make opinion-driven decisions about vaccines, which leads to disease outbreaks, negatively impacting their health and the health of others. These differences between public opinion and public health data demonstrate that the context of preexisting community beliefs matters. In fact, beliefs are often held sacred. As humans, we are naturally more inclined to look for data, however flimsy, that support these beliefs and rebut any data, however sound, that threaten to topple them.

The disease and death linked to opinion-driven health behaviors represent serious public health concerns that could be averted if public health data communication was routinely successful. Our contention in this chapter is that data are a powerful tool in shaping health policy, but their power for positive change in our communities is diminished because too often we refuse to listen to one other. At times, it seems public health officials and community members are entangled in a bitter divorce with irreconcilable differences. There has been a breakdown in communication, so when public health officials say, for example, "vaccines are safe and prevent diseases," segments of the community surmise only that these public health officials are lying and cannot be trusted. Communicating more public health data will do nothing to correct this stalemate. So, what will? Before we propose an approach for finding common ground, consider a second case example, which is important for context.

Case #2: Evidence-Based Versus Community Voice

The co-sleeping case example is just one illustration of the common tension between scientific evidence and community opinion. A second example comes from Healthy Start, a national program to improve perinatal outcomes and reduce disparities. Healthy Start was launched in the early 1990s and is now located in over 100 US cities where infant mortality is higher than the national average.[6] Healthy Start programs offer an array of services based on the individual needs of each participant that are shaped through a community consortium. The community consortium includes residents who seek to identify and fill gaps that may negatively impact local health outcomes. For this reason, Healthy Start is an exemplar of public health practice including community will in the equation when designing initiatives.

Because each Healthy Start site tailors its services based on community voice, the exact array of services differs across sites. They are uniquely responsive to community needs and input. However, all Healthy Start programs have a community-based steering committee and a case management and home visitation component. Healthy Start program leaders and advocates believe their approach to home visiting, which has been in operation for over three decades, is among the best with excellent health improvement outcomes. Scientific evaluators, on the other hand, see it differently. In fact, evaluators find it challenging—even impossible—to evaluate the effectiveness of Healthy Start home visiting efforts for several reasons. First, variations across Healthy Start home visiting programs are substantial, and while variations like these can be accounted for in evaluation models, without careful data collection they can limit the ability to definitively assess program impact. Second, Healthy Start sites have not emphasized routine and standardized data collection. Consequently, little consistent data has been available across sites. Finally, the Healthy Start program is not conducted like a clinical trial. Instead, all participants receive the interventions (i.e., no randomization) and opt in freely at widely variable stages of pregnancy. These factors inhibit cohort comparisons to other similar groups who did not receive the Healthy Start home visiting intervention.

The disagreement about the effectiveness of Healthy Start's approach to home visiting came to a head when the Affordable Care Act (ACA) became law and a new infusion of funding for home visiting was initialized through the Maternal, Infant, and Early Childhood Home Visiting Program.[7] Those receiving funds were mandated to choose from a preapproved list of evidence-based home visiting programs, which had been vetted by the Department of Health and Human Services. When Healthy Start advocates first heard of this review process, they anticipated their home visiting model would rise to the top. Having witnessed, and in many cases personally experienced, the positive impacts of the program, they were eager to see these new and substantial federal dollars help spread and scale their model to thousands of additional families across the country. Their hopes were reasonable. After all, Healthy Start program participants generally belong to sociodemographic groups who experience infant mortality rates twice the national average, and all Healthy Start sites are in communities experiencing at least 1.5 times the national infant mortality average; however, Healthy Start program participants have a demonstrated and longstanding infant mortality rate well below the national average.[8] As one report issued by the National Healthy Start Association in response to ACA passage described,

> The federal Healthy Start Initiative, with its cost-effective, community-driven model of care, has a major role to play in the historic Health Affordable Care Act (ACA) Maternal, Infant and Early Childhood Home Visiting Program's national efforts to build quality, comprehensive statewide early childhood systems for pregnant women, parents, caregivers and children from birth to eight years. The 104 federal Healthy Start sites are "shovel ready" to assist in improving quality of health care, enhancing disease prevention and strengthening the health care workforce.[9(p3)]

Unfortunately for all those who believed in the power of Healthy Start and its community-based approach to tailoring home visiting services, federal officials responsible for overseeing ACA implementation were not convinced. The official federal website notes only the following in relation to the program: "HHS has determined that Healthy Start is not eligible for review... because it is a federal grant program and not a home visiting model. Information on Healthy Start has been removed from the website."[10]

Nearly a decade after ACA implementation, tensions continue to run high between federal officials and Healthy Start advocates. Many Healthy Start advocates are former program participants who benefited greatly from the program and now dedicate their time to helping other families. Early in the ACA's implementation, the authors attended a national conference and witnessed a public exchange between the federal officials running the new ACA Home Visiting program and multiple Healthy Start advocates. Following a panel presentation detailing the process used to assess home visiting evidence and select the approved programs, Healthy Start advocates lined up at the microphones. The presenters were likely expecting—even hoping—to field nuanced questions about their assessment methodology. Instead, one by one, the Healthy Start advocates shared their compelling and deeply personal pleas for inclusion of Healthy Start among the approved list of programs. The advocates' words were filled with passion and a fair amount of outrage that the list seemed to be dominated by programs developed by researchers and academicians far removed from the realities they had personally lived. Through it all, however, the federal officials remained stoic and unwavering in their final assessment. Since that time, additional approved programs have been added to the list, but Healthy Start remains excluded.

This case example raises a key question: What is evidence? Further, why aren't our definitions of evidence all the same? No doubt when the Healthy Start advocates were telling their individual stories of program impact—how participation in the program had resulted in a full-term healthy birth when all the signs pointed the other direction—they believed what they were sharing was rock-solid evidence. But the federal officials on stage found it easy to dismiss these testimonials as little more than anecdotes. The federal officials were equally perplexed by why their carefully crafted presentations, transparently outlining their entire analytic approach, did not seem to silence objections. It was genuinely confusing why their math didn't compute with the audience. In fact, during the exchange, a federal official tried to respond by questioning if the Healthy Start advocate at the microphone had heard his presentation. The audience immediately erupted in shock and boos. He quickly tried to backpedal, stammering something about his question being sincere and that it was not intended as an insult. His backpedal showed something interesting in his thinking: the only reasonable response when faced with his thorough and accurately conducted scientific analysis was simply to agree. In his mind, the audience member must have arrived late or stepped out to take a call. That had to be the case because if she had been present, she would certainly acquiesce. No doubt the Healthy Start advocates were similarly baffled as to why their testimonials had no impact. Data are all too often seen as a decider when they are really a starting point for conversation.

FINDING COMMON GROUND

The examples provided in this chapter lead us to ask, What is at the crux of these disagreements and how do we find common ground? Understanding these things is critical if we are going to be effective at using public health data.

When considering what is at the crux of the disagreement, it might be easy to presume that arguments like these boil down to the difference between words and numbers. Perhaps some of it can be attributed to that. After all, people do tend to gravitate toward one or the other: "I'm a numbers guy" or opposingly, "I love a good story." But we shouldn't be so quick to reduce the evidence debate to words versus numbers, nor should we accept a simplistic dichotomy between words and numbers. Both are valuable. Both are necessary. The Healthy Start case example illustrates how all sides in any public health debate are telling stories carefully crafted to be as convincing as possible. Some may lean more heavily on numbers than others, but all the stories are crafted to shape what counts as truth. The authors contend that the most convincing and accurate of these stories will be the ones that contain personal experiences and in-depth data analysis.

If the difference is not as simple as words versus numbers, perhaps it is about differing ideologies concerning how government programs should be run. A political debate. Here again, there is a case to be made because public health programs are often initiated by elected officials and imbued with their party's political ideologies. Healthy Start, for example, was created under the George W. Bush administration and designed to promote flexibility. Historically, Republican administrations shunned what they viewed as heavy-handed government intervention in the lives of citizens. Healthy Start fits well with this philosophy, giving autonomy to local programs to shape and reshape what they believe is needed and will work for them locally. The ACA, on the other hand, was developed under the Barack Obama administration and, rather than working to keep government's touch light, it sought comprehensive solutions that would fundamentally change health care access, affordability, and quality for all Americans.

Regardless of one's political leanings, it is fair to acknowledge that these aims differ dramatically, and due to constant flip-flopping of legislative and executive leadership at the local, state, and federal levels, we are left with a patchwork of mismatched public health programs. When it comes to home visiting, the passage of the ACA has resulted in the power and money being amassed on the side that, ironically, is known as Taylorism. At the end of the nineteenth century in the industrializing United States, Frederick Winslow Taylor developed the theory of Scientific Management.[11] Taylor believed there was one right way. More specifically, he believed we could use empirical observation to discover the truth about workplace efficiencies—the best way to dig a hole, carry a heavy object, inspect a ball bearing, or assemble an automobile (Henry Ford's moving assembly line might be the most iconic example of Taylorism). Taylor's theory resonated, changing the way we view the workplace and how management prescribes how tasks must be completed, when, by whom, and for what compensation. Taylor's ideas and Ford's methods were adopted in Japan as well during the reconstruction following World War II. There, they resulted in the development of advanced quality control methods and greater autonomy to employees to observe processes and propose improvements. Over one hundred years later, his devotees in public health—none of whom likely know his name—still ascribe to Scientific Management and hold that empirical observation should be used to discover the best way to do everything, including home visits.

Opponents of this perspective view public health more like Muhammad Ali viewed boxing. When Ali was asked why his style changed from one fight to the next, he responded simply, "I got different strokes for different folks."[12] From that interview, Ali's clever turn of phrase became a "truth" that resonated. Sly and the Family Stone used it as lyrics in their hit song "Everyday People" and the popular ABC sitcom *Different Strokes* was named in honor of the expression. Ali even had a cameo on the show. Taylor would have insisted there was one best way to box, but it's hard to argue with Ali's results in the ring.

Rather than continuing to beat one another up, how can the two sides come together and agree on needed public health actions?

TOWARD MORE CONSENSUS IN PUBLIC HEALTH DECISION MAKING

Whether these differences stem from personal affinity for words or numbers, preferences in how government should be run, or any other source, our goal should be to find value in our differences. It may be overly ambitious to believe we can settle all debates about what public health actions are needed, when they should be taken, or how exactly we should carry them out. Instead, our best hope may be to train public health leaders to have strong social and emotional skills as they engage the public in using data to inform our public health actions. At present, very little of the academic preparation for public health professionals focuses on these skills. However, as we have seen from the examples in this chapter, competence in understanding ourselves and others and responding in ways that demonstrate empathy and lead to shared trust could make all the difference when using data to inform public health practice.

These abilities are grounded in what is known as emotional intelligence. Beginning in 1990, scholars first separated emotional intelligence as a unique form of intelligence distinct from previously accepted standards of intellect.[13] Across the ensuing decade, multiple models of emotional intelligence were developed, often for different purposes (e.g., business and leadership, neurological research), but generally these models shared similar domains. One particularly useful model was developed by Daniel Goleman and includes the four domains of self-awareness, self-management, social awareness, and relationship management (Table 4-1).[1] In the following sections, we provide an overview of how public

Table 4-1. Emotional Intelligence Domains and Associated Competencies

Self-Awareness	Social Awareness
• *Emotional self-awareness*: Reading one's own emotions and recognizing their impact; using "gut sense" to guide decisions • *Accurate self-assessment*: Knowing one's strengths and limits • *Self-confidence*: A sound sense of one's self-worth and capabilities • ***Key data use skill***: Take time to assess how specific aspects of public health data personally resonate with you	• *Empathy*: Sensing others' emotions, understanding their perspectives, and taking active interest in their concerns • *Organizational awareness*: Reading the currents, decision networks, and politics at the organizational level • *Service*: Recognizing and meeting follower, client, or customer needs • ***Key data use skill***: Take time to assess how specific aspects of public health data might be received by others who think differently than you
Self-Management	**Relationship Management**
• *Emotional self-control*: Keeping disruptive emotions and impulses under control • *Transparency*: Displaying honesty and integrity; trustworthiness • *Adaptability*: Flexibility in adapting to changing situations or overcoming obstacles • *Achievement*: The drive to improve performance to meet inner standards of excellence • *Initiative*: Readiness to act and seize opportunities • *Optimism*: Seeing the upside in events • ***Key data use skill***: Always remain open to considering new public health data and fresh analytic interpretations of the data	• *Inspirational leadership*: Guiding and motivating with a compelling vision • *Influence*: Wielding a range of tactics for persuasion • *Developing others*: Bolstering others' abilities through feedback and guidance • *Change catalyst*: Initiating, managing, and leading in a new direction • *Conflict management*: Resolving disagreements • *Building bonds*: Cultivating and maintaining a web of relationships • *Teamwork and collaboration*: Cooperation and team building • ***Key data use skill***: Use public health data as a conversation starter rather than seeing it as the final decider

Source: Based on Goleman et al.[1]

health leaders could best apply the emotional intelligence model as they work with data and community members to build consensus and reach decisions on needed actions.

Self-Awareness

In the emotional intelligence framework, self-awareness is defined as having a "deep understanding of one's emotions, as well as one's strengths and limitations and one's values and motives."[1(p40)] When applied specifically to using data to build consensus for public health action, the importance of self-awareness cannot be understated. The key data use skill here is to take time to assess how specific aspects of public health data personally resonate with you.

In Chapter 1 of this book, we introduced the positionality exercise and each of the authors shared their personal positionality statements. The positionality exercise can serve as an excellent foundation for a comprehensive, initial self-awareness examination.

It allows us to better understand our core values and how our lived experience has helped shape what we hold most important. Understanding our positionality also allows us to more easily assess our emotional responses to events in the moment by providing us with the equivalent of a diagnostic checklist.

To remain self-aware in your work with data, especially the more collaborative aspects such as presenting data and collectively using it to shape public health action, consider the following practical activities.

- **Develop and routinely revisit your positionality statement.** Staying current with your positionality allows you to stay grounded in your core values and not get lost or distracted by the details. Public health leaders who are sure of their positionality can stay focused on the big picture and remain committed to a shared vision of better health for all. Interestingly, we have found that a strong and current connection to our positionality ultimately leads to better relationship management and more effective collaboration.
- **Schedule time to conduct self-assessments during data collection and analysis, especially prior to data sharing.** Few of us are intentional about routinely conducting self-assessments. However, when it comes to working with data to examine and improve the health of communities, we should view it as a responsibility. Doing so can help ensure our intentions are correctly aligned with the communities most directly impacted by the health issues we are considering and might enable us to glimpse the possible impact the numbers will have on others.

Self-Management

Being aware of our emotions is essential but is only the first step. To effectively guide community groups in thoughtful analysis of data for action, public health leaders must also be able to manage stress, anxiety, and other emotions that could be counterproductive and potentially harmful to group cohesion. Strong emotional responses can be common when dealing with sensitive issues related to the health of our communities and when working with groups that are likely to have members who disagree with our perspectives. Left unchecked, these powerful emotions will have an impact on others, often producing reciprocal negative responses.[1] The key data use skill here is to always remain open to considering new public health data and fresh analytic interpretations of the data. In fact, as individuals who deeply value public health data and their analysis, we should be interested consumers of new data and interpretations. This does not mean that we accept every new analysis we encounter, but immediately dismissing data because they appear to contradict our existing perspectives is an emotional reaction rather than a scientific perspective.

With all this discussion concerning emotions, it is important to point out that emotions are an essential and beautiful aspect of our human and social existence. The work of emotional intelligence is not meant to stifle emotions in ourselves or others. Rather, the aim is to be cognizant of their existence and impact and harness their power for our collective advantage. As effective public health data users, consider the following activities to practice effective self-management.

- **Place a high value on community data deliberation.** It can be easy to fall into the trap of valuing only the end result of deliberation. Beyond that, sometimes it is tempting to exclusively value an end result that is to our liking. However, deliberativeness is a democratic value just like inclusivity or equality. Leading community groups through a lively, engaged, and even, at times, contentious deliberation about health outcomes and potential strategies for improvement should drive us as public health professionals. Deliberation means our data are being heard and having an impact.
- **Be willing to offer your perspective on action without being authoritative.** Aligned with valuing community data deliberation, optimal self-management can be easier to attain when we strive for humility when sharing our opinions. Try expressing your perspective about how the data speak to possible public health actions and then listening to find out if your sentiments resonate with others. Avoid speaking in collective imperatives such as "we must." Instead, express personal values using phrases that begin with "I feel" or "it is important to me."
- **Remain flexible and open-minded, willing to compromise or accept the will of the majority.** Without question, this can be a challenge, especially when we feel passionate about the health of our community—as we should—and believe the available data indicate a different course of action. Compromise does not mean we are ignoring the science and data. It simply means that after giving it our all to collect, analyze, interpret, and present the data, we are willing to accept the will of the democratic majority. They saw the same data, but somehow, they saw it differently or came to a different consensus about what to do in light of the data. When this happens, we as public health professionals do not write off the dissenting community voice as irrational, unscientific, or any other derogative. Instead, we redouble our efforts to understand their position, reexamine our own, and use data to the best of our ability to inform public health decision making. It can also be reassuring to remember that public health actions are never once-and-for-all solutions. It would be great if they were, but unfortunately, population health promotion requires constant vigilance and ongoing action. If the solution you thought best was not the will of the majority, you can support the consensus decision while continuing to humbly advance your proposal and looking for the next implementation opportunity. Chances are, it will come around again soon and hopefully we have laid the groundwork for it with our previous efforts rather than burned possible bridges.

Social Awareness

Social awareness is the first of the domains that moves us from personal to interpersonal. Goleman and colleagues stress the importance of empathy, noting it as "the fundamental competence of social awareness."[1(p50)] Empathy allows us to perceive the emotional responses of others and perhaps even grasp the *why* behind emotions. The key data use skill here is to take time to assess how specific aspects of public health data might be received by others who think differently than you.

Social awareness for public health professionals also involves a good deal of political perception—a unique subset of social awareness. Health decisions that impact the voting public can quickly become politically charged. Being able to predict these instances and navigate smoothly through contentious issues requires social acumen and awareness. To remain socially aware while using data to inform public health action, consider the following strategies.

- **Consider who is impacted by the data.** Public health professionals deal with data every day. As such, it can be easy for us to become calloused to its impact and not consider who the data might affect. Stepping back from our data familiarity and attempting to view it from a fresh perspective and through the eyes of others is a valuable exercise. As stewards of the public's health, we should strive to understand and relate to the perspectives of all constituents in our communities.
- **Build meaningful relationships.** Effectively practicing the previous point—relating the perspectives of others—becomes less of an abstract exercise when we build meaningful relationships. Getting to know and care about the members of our community allows us to understand more readily how certain health issues and policy responses would be received by them. Public health leaders should endeavor to build a broad and diverse network and actively seek out the perspectives of network members as they go about their work.
- **Be mindful of power and politics.** Effective public health professionals will consider which body is most likely—and most appropriate—to make decisions about the data. We may want an invested community group to have ownership over a policy that will affect them. This is an honorable aim. However, if that policy is currently a hot topic in the state legislature, it is unlikely the community group will have that opportunity. In these situations, it remains important to communicate openly with all impacted groups, while being honest about the power and politics at play. When the opportunity arises, it is also valuable to be ready with the data and the voices of community members to share with elected officials and others who have decision making authority.

Relationship Management

The final domain of emotional intelligence can be viewed as the culmination of the previous three. Relationship management involves a diverse set of skills, timed and applied to properly fit the context. Self-awareness, self-management, and social awareness are the prerequisites for getting relationship management right. Does the situation call for an impassioned plea or conflict management? Alternatively, is deep listening the best response? Expert relationship managers will have an accurate sense of what is needed and a practiced approach to effectively bringing that to the social exchange. The key data use skill here is learning to use public health data as a conversation starter rather than seeing it as the final decider. To use data effectively and help communities act upon it, the following relationship management activities are important.

- **Use the positionality exercise with others.** Using the positionality exercise with groups (along with other smaller self-awareness activities) can be immensely helpful. Being grounded in our own positionality is important, but imagine the power of an entire collaborative group knowing their own and one another's positionality. This work builds understanding and trust between members. Even when disagreements arise over what the data mean or what actions should be taken in response to the data, this effort up front makes it easier to see the perspectives of others and come to common ground.
- **Think small, but persistent.** There is an old expression that reminds us that "the force of the waves is in their persistence." Too often, we seek sweeping changes that we hope and believe will mightily correct an adverse health outcome. The challenge is that such changes are incredibly hard to build support around, let alone implement and sustain. Even when implementation occurs, these large-scale efforts often fail to realize the substantial gains we had envisioned. Pursuing multiple smaller decisions can often have strategic value. When groups see they were successful at deliberating on the data, coming to consensus, and implementing a response, they can become intoxicated with that process, engaging it again and again in iterative actions to consistently improve their community's health.

SUMMARY

In this chapter, we provided real-world examples of times when public health decision making was challenging and involved significant conflict. Data can be a powerful tool in guiding the decisions we make and believe are necessary to achieve better health for all members of our community. However, the use of data is a skill that stretches beyond collection and analysis to involve emotional intelligence. In the hands of adept, emotionally intelligent public health leaders, data can clarify goals, suggest needed strategies, prompt action, and even instill passion and fortitude for the sustained effort that is often needed to realize improvements in population health. To help public health professionals use data with greater emotional intelligence, this chapter presented four key data use skills: (1) take time to assess how specific aspects of public health data personally resonate with you; (2) always remain open to considering new public health data and fresh analytic interpretations of the data; (3) take time to assess how specific aspects of public health data might be received by others who think differently than you; and (4) use public health data as a conversation starter rather than seeing it as the final decider.

As we conclude this chapter, take a moment to consider the two case examples provided in earlier sections. If you were in those situations or similar situations in the future, what would you do differently? Which of your core values would be most pertinent to those circumstances? Would finding common ground be possible, and would that common ground improve, or perhaps diminish the effectiveness of the public health activities selected? As a final reflection, which of the domains of emotional intelligence—self-awareness, self-management, social awareness, or relationship management—do you think these cases reveal as most critical when using data to inform public health action?

REFERENCES

1. Goleman D, Boyatzis RE, McKee A. *Primal Leadership: Unleashing the Power of Emotional Intelligence.* Harvard Business Review Press; 2013.
2. Goleman, D. Emotional intelligence: Issues in paradigm building. In: Cherniss C, Goleman D, eds. *The Emotionally Intelligent Workplace: How to Select for, Measure, and Improve Emotional Intelligence in Individuals, Groups, and Organizations.* Jossey-Bass; 2001:13–26.
3. Hanlon JJ. Is there a future for local health departments? *Health Serv Rep.* 1973;88(10):898–901. doi:10.2307/4594951
4. D'Arcy J. Co-sleeping with butcher knives: Are these Milwaukee PSAs overkill? *Washington Post.* November 21, 2011. Accessed April 2, 2024. https://www.washingtonpost.com/blogs/on-parenting/post/co-sleeping-with-butcher-knives-are-these-milwaukee-psas-overkill/2011/11/16/gIQA7tmKiN_blog.html
5. Llorens I. Controversial co-sleeping ad features baby next to knife. *HuffPost.* November 16, 2011. Accessed April 2, 2024. https://www.huffpost.com/entry/co-sleeping-ad-baby-knife-dangers_n_1097170
6. Health Resources and Services Administration. Healthy Start: Nurturing health, preventing disparities. Accessed April 2, 2025. https://mchb.hrsa.gov/programs-impact/healthy-start
7. Health Resources and Services Administration. Maternal, Infant, and Early Childhood Home Visiting (MIECHV) Program. Accessed April 2, 2024. https://mchb.hrsa.gov/programs-impact/programs/home-visiting/maternal-infant-early-childhood-home-visiting-miechv-program
8. National Healthy Start Association. Accessed April 2, 2024. https://www.nationalhealthystart.org

9. Berry E, Brady C, Cunningham SD, et al. *Federal Healthy Start Initiative: A National Network for Effective Home Visitation and Family Support Services.* National Healthy Start Association; 2010. Accessed April 2, 2024. https://www.nationalhealthystart.org/wp-content/uploads/2021/04/NHSA_WhitePaper.pdf
10. US Dept of Health and Human Services. Healthy Start-Home Visiting. Home Visiting Evidence of Effectiveness. Accessed April 2, 2024. https://homvee.acf.hhs.gov/models/healthy-start-home-visiting
11. Taylor FW. *The Principles of Scientific Management.* Harper & Brothers; 1919.
12. Reed B. Muhammad Ali's best quotes: 'Float like a butterfly, sting like a bee.' *The Guardian.* June 4, 2016. Accessed April 2, 2024. https://www.theguardian.com/sport/2016/jun/04/muhammad-ali-greatest-quotes-sting-butterfly-louisville-lip
13. Cherniss C, Goleman D, eds. *The Emotionally Intelligent Workplace: How to Select for, Measure, and Improve Emotional Intelligence in Individuals, Groups, and Organizations.* Jossey-Bass; 2001.

Conclusion: Better Access to Essential Data

Data-informed decision making is at the heart of effective public health practice. As we have explored throughout this book, the ability to leverage diverse data sources is necessary for activities such as surveillance, evaluation, quality improvement, needs assessment, and program planning. However, in the authors' experience, restrictions on data access and use often cause excessive delays or even prevent health departments from fulfilling these core data functions. Many health departments report that these challenges have increased in recent years.

As a nation, the epidemiological capacity of our health departments is far from adequate to perform basic public health services.[1] To fill temporary gaps caused by turnover, or even as a permanent staffing solution, health departments (especially local, tribal, and territorial health departments) often rely on outside organizations, such as hospital systems, nonprofits, and academic partners. Though the Health Insurance Portability and Accountability Act (HIPAA) Privacy Rule allows public health authorities to use data that include personal health information,[2] the involvement of outside organizations may introduce legal and data security concerns, leading to further restrictions. In some states, staffing shortages have also delayed the processing and dissemination of core public health data files and summary data reports.

We acknowledge the necessity of data protection and privacy measures. Restrictions help ensure that data about individuals are handled in ways that assure security and confidentiality. Security is not the only issue that data owners and users may be concerned about. They share the responsibility to ensure that data are analyzed correctly, using appropriate statistical methods. In addition, there may be legitimate concerns around the dissemination of findings, including community and political sensitivities. Responsible data use requires that these concerns be addressed.

Yet, the reality is that lack of access to data has far-reaching consequences. It hampers the ability of health departments and their partners to make informed decisions based on the best available evidence. It prevents the use of data collected, processed, and maintained at taxpayer expense. Ultimately, it impacts the health and well-being of communities.

Thankfully, there are solutions and funding mechanisms in place to support some of the solutions.[3] For example, federal and philanthropic funding supports training, including university-based degree and certification programs, post-degree work experiences, and both on-demand training modules and in-person training experiences for epidemiologists who are already working in the field. Additionally, the Centers for Disease

Control and Prevention (CDC) has recognized the need to modernize the technology infrastructure and make different data sources more compatible and useful. Data modernization efforts such as these are taking place across the globe. As this move toward a great emphasis on data modernization and use takes place, it is essential that we ensure standards of data justice are established and utilized.[4] Data justice aims to ensure comprehensive fairness in the way data are handled and used, paying particular attention to how representative the data are to all populations, how well privacy is protected, how open access is permitted, who owns the data, and to what degree the benefits of data use are equally distributed across society. As we increasingly improve and modernize our ability to use data to inform all kinds of policy, we must simultaneously champion a call for improved data justice.

Despite these ongoing efforts, data systems do not yet allow for easy linkage and sharing in many places, and demand for training opportunities outstrips availability. Progress in data sharing will likely require that standards for data security be developed, codified, taught, and incorporated into legislation at all levels, and CDC efforts are supporting these goals.[5] Data use agreements must consider that many public health practitioners are not part of government health departments. Formal partnership agreements between governmental and nongovernmental practitioners may be needed. Training in privacy and data security requirements, like the Collaborative Institutional Training Initiative's research training, should be created for public health data managers and analysts to support core functions. The requirements will likely be quite different, due to the public health need for rapid response to emerging threats, ongoing standardized surveillance, and often very localized planning, quality improvement, and program evaluation.

To more efficiently meet the training needs of health departments, it will be important to include local and state practitioners in planning. High turnover and understaffing present challenges. Often, epidemiologists in health departments are trained in one area but find themselves serving in another, or in several areas. Therefore, they may have a strong foundation in general epidemiologic methods but lack specialized knowledge of data sources and methods in some areas for which they are responsible, increasing the risk of methodological errors. More opportunities for rapid onboarding in specific areas may be needed. Mentoring relationships and increased networking opportunities for people using specific data sources or working on specific health problems might multiply the impact of existing on-demand training resources.

Ultimately, we must meet both needs: safeguarding data privacy and enabling the responsible and effective use of data for the betterment of public health. By fostering open dialogues, establishing clear guidelines, and promoting collaboration among stakeholders, we can pave the way for a future where data-informed decision making becomes the norm, empowering communities and driving meaningful improvements in population health outcomes.

REFERENCES

1. Arrazola J, Auer S. Assessment of epidemiology capacity in state health departments — United States, 2021. *MMWR Morb Mortal Wkly Rep.* 2022;71:484–488. doi:10.15585/mmwr.mm7113a2
2. US Dept of Health and Human Services, Office for Civil Rights. Disclosures for Public Health Activities. Revised April 3, 2003. Accessed May 1, 2024. https://www.hhs.gov/hipaa/for-professionals/privacy/guidance/disclosures-public-health-activities/index.html
3. Centers for Disease Control and Prevention. About the Public Health Data Strategy. Updated January 16, 2025. Accessed February 16, 2025. https://www.cdc.gov/public-health-data-strategy/php/about/index.html
4. Heeks R, Shekhar S. Datafication, development and marginalised urban communities: An applied data justice framework. *Inf Commun Soc.* 2019;22(7):992–1011. doi:10.1080/1369118X.2019.1599039
5. Centers for Disease Control and Prevention. 2022 Data Modernization Initiative snapshot. April 22, 2024. Accessed May 2, 2024. https://www.cdc.gov/surveillance/data-modernization/snapshot/2022-snapshot/index.html

About the Authors

Chad Abresch, PhD is the Weitz family chair of health promotion and department chair in the College of Public Health at the University of Nebraska Medical Center (UNMC). With over two decades of leadership in maternal and child health, he has spearheaded innovative public health programs and partnerships that have improved health outcomes nationwide. His work focuses on community-engaged solutions to address persistent public health challenges in the United States. Abresch also serves as principal investigator and senior advisor for CityMatCH, a national organization strengthening public health leaders to improve the health of women, families, and communities.

Carol Gilbert, PhD, MS is an assistant professor in the Department of Health Promotion at UNMC's College of Public Health, where she also serves as senior health data analyst for CityMatCH. Her work focuses on empowering communities to effectively use local data and research findings for public health planning and decision making. Gilbert's expertise includes analyzing the impact of data quality problems on preventable mortality estimates and applying frameworks and methods to help communities translate epidemiologic surveillance findings into meaningful policy change and public health action.

Regina Idoate, PhD is a mother, educator, social creative, citizen of the Cherokee Nation, and community-engaged Indigenous health researcher who serves as associate professor and director of spirituality, culture, and health in the College of Public Health at UNMC. Her research focuses on community systems in relation to culture and ecology, with particular interest in maternal and child health. She works to create opportunities to weave modern science and Indigenous knowledge with local context to promote Indigenous health innovations in community-based settings. Her active research centers Indigenous health and education in medical humanities, workforce development, and community-driven social innovation. Idoate wants to promote healthier future generations in ways that respect and celebrate Indigenous People, culture, and land, and to do this with a teachable spirit. She collaborates across disciplines and cultures and appreciates time and space to play, pray, wonder, and wander in kinship with all our relations.

Ellen (El) Kerns, PhD, MPH is an assistant professor in the Division of Health System Sciences in the Department of Pediatrics in the College of Medicine at UNMC. She has several operational and research director roles within UNMC, regionally with the Great Plains Clinical Translational Research Network, and nationally with the American Academy of Pediatrics, with a common focus on ensuring that data becomes actionable information for patients, caregivers, researchers, health care providers, and public health organizations. She utilizes her combined expertise in clinical informatics, public health, and statistics to leverage health information resources and technologies to improve the lives of children, families, and communities.

Aislinn Rookwood, PhD is an assistant professor in the Department of Health Promotion in the College of Public Health at UNMC. Her work focuses on utilizing community-driven approaches, workforce development, and health promotion theory to reduce disparities in maternal and child health, particularly in children's environmental health, and cancer prevention efforts. At the heart of this work, she aims to collaborate with communities to address health disparities and advance health equity.

Index

Page numbers followed by *b* and *f* indicate boxes and figures, respectively.

M

N

O

P